Living w

'The problem of IBS often extends far beyond ... every area of one's life, an issue that can be missed by many healthcare providers. I am pleased to say that this issue is not missed in the book you hold in your hands. Rather, Drs Ferreira and Gillanders have produced something that specifically aims to help people suffering from IBS achieve a life that is less restricted by IBS; a life that also has meaning, vitality and quality. I have no doubt that the approach in this book will allow better living with IBS.'

> — **Kevin E. Vowles, PhD, Consultant Clinical Psychologist,**
> **The Haywood Hospital**

'This is a very worthwhile book for people who suffer from the unpleasant symptoms of Irritable Bowel Syndrome. Once the reader has been given an overview to this condition they are introduced to a range of workable ways to deal with it. Packed with practical exercises and scenarios, *Better Living with IBS* helps people to live the way that they want, potentially improving their overall quality of life. I would highly recommend this easily accessed text to anyone with IBS and to all health professions who deal with this complex chronic condition.'

> — **Dr Graeme D. Smith, University of Edinburgh**

Overcoming Common Problems Series

Selected titles

A full list of titles is available from Sheldon Press,
36 Causton Street, London SW1P 4ST and on our website at
www.sheldonpress.co.uk

101 Questions to Ask Your Doctor
Dr Tom Smith

Birth Over 35
Sheila Kitzinger

Bulimia, Binge-eating and their Treatment
Professor J. Hubert Lacey, Dr Bryony Bamford
and Amy Brown

Coeliac Disease: What you need to know
Alex Gazzola

Coping Successfully with Shyness
Margaret Oakes, Professor Robert Bor
and Dr Carina Eriksen

Coping with Anaemia
Dr Tom Smith

Coping with Asthma in Adults
Mark Greener

Coping with Bronchitis and Emphysema
Dr Tom Smith

Coping with Drug Problems in the Family
Lucy Jolin

Coping with Dyspraxia
Jill Eckersley

Coping with Early-onset Dementia
Jill Eckersley

Coping with Envy
Dr Windy Dryden

Coping with Gout
Christine Craggs-Hinton

**Coping with Manipulation: When others
blame you for their feelings**
Dr Windy Dryden

**Coping with Obsessive Compulsive
Disorder**
Professor Kevin Gournay, Rachel Piper
and Professor Paul Rogers

Coping with Stomach Ulcers
Dr Tom Smith

Depressive Illness: The curse of the strong
Dr Tim Cantopher

**Divorce and Separation: A legal guide
for all couples**
Dr Mary Welstead

Dying for a Drink
Dr Tim Cantopher

**Epilepsy: Complementary and alternative
treatments**
Dr Sallie Baxendale

The Heart Attack Survival Guide
Mark Greener

High-risk Body Size: Take control of your weight
Dr Funké Baffour

How to Beat Worry and Stress
Dr David Delvin

How to Develop Inner Strength
Dr Windy Dryden

**Let's Stay Together: A guide to lasting
relationships**
Jane Butterworth

Living with IBS
Nuno Ferreira and David T. Gillanders

**Living with a Problem Drinker:
Your survival guide**
Rolande Anderson

Living with Tinnitus and Hyperacusis
Dr Laurence McKenna, Dr David Baguley
and Dr Don McFerran

Losing a Parent
Fiona Marshall

Making Sense of Trauma: How to tell your story
Dr Nigel C. Hunt and Dr Sue McHale

Motor Neurone Disease: A family affair
Dr David Oliver

Natural Treatments for Arthritis
Christine Craggs-Hinton

**Overcoming Gambling: A guide for problem
and compulsive gamblers**
Philip Mawer

Overcoming Loneliness
Alice Muir

**The Pain Management Handbook:
Your personal guide**
Neville Shone

Reducing Your Risk of Dementia
Dr Tom Smith

**Therapy for Beginners: How to get the best
out of counselling**
Professor Robert Bor, Sheila Gill and Anne Stokes

**Transforming Eight Deadly Emotions
into Healthy Ones**
Dr Windy Dryden

Treating Arthritis: The drug-free way
Margaret Hills and Christine Horner

Treating Arthritis: The supplements guide
Julia Davies

Overcoming Common Problems

Living with IBS

NUNO FERREIRA, PhD
DR DAVID T. GILLANDERS (CPsychol)

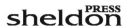

Originally published in Australia in 2012 as
*Better Living with IBS: A step-by-step program to managing
your symptoms so you can enjoy life to the full!* by
Exisle Publishing Pty Ltd, Wollombi, New South Wales, Australia,
and Auckland, New Zealand

First published in Great Britain in 2012

Sheldon Press
36 Causton Street
London SW1P 4ST
www.sheldonpress.co.uk

British Library Cataloguing-in-Publication Data
A catalogue record for this book is available from the British Library

ISBN 978-1-84709-250-2
eBook ISBN 978-1-84709-251-9

Typeset by Fakenham Prepress Solutions, Fakenham, Norfolk NR21 8NN
Printed in Great Britain by Ashford Colour Press
Subsequently digitally printed in Great Britain

Produced on paper from sustainable forests

Contents

The tables and boxes in this book are for guidance only and can be copied and used as a starting point, either as they are or adapted to your own particular purpose. Feel free to take a piece of paper and write as much as you like.

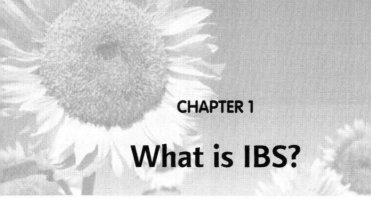

CHAPTER 1

What is IBS?

You are not alone

If you are reading this book you are part of a large community of people who have to deal with the difficult condition known as Irritable Bowel Syndrome (IBS) on a daily basis. An estimated 10–20 per cent of the population living in the Western world is affected by symptoms that would constitute a diagnosis of Irritable Bowel Syndrome — in fact, so many people present with IBS that some specialists have called it the common cold of the gastrointestinal illnesses.

In this book — and particularly this chapter — we will review some basic information about IBS. You might feel that you already have a sound knowledge (and experience) of IBS, and some patients are indeed experts about their condition. If you are part of this group, we invite you to just keep reading and review or refresh the information you already have. On the other hand, you might feel that you don't have enough information about your condition or that you are unsure about some aspects of it; in this case we encourage you to carefully read the information in this chapter.

The abundance of information about IBS from a wide range of sources can cause confusion and lead to inaccuracies, so we want you to have a good understanding of what IBS is before we proceed with our approach to living with the condition. Throughout this book we will provide you with a comprehensive program supported by exercises that will help you find ways to live a successful life while managing your IBS.

Also, we understand that reading about IBS might bring up some uncomfortable feelings or thoughts. This is perfectly natural and will be the focus of our next chapter. For now, we ask you to stay with that discomfort and go through the chapter at your own pace. Finally, and before we begin, we would like you to think a bit about the following question: How would you rate your everyday distress related to IBS right now? If 1 were 'I am distress-free' and 10 were 'I am extremely distressed', which would you be?

We'll return to this estimate later in this chapter. But now, let's focus on the basics of Irritable Bowel Syndrome.

Introducing IBS — a functional disorder

IBS is part of a group of disorders called functional disorders. A functional disorder is a physical illness that cannot be explained by organic disease or by a demonstrable structural or biochemical change. What this means is that this type of disorder causes symptoms without any visible disease process or tissue damage. This does not mean that the symptoms are not real; what it means is that doctors cannot see anything wrong or changed in the organ or system that accounts for its malfunction. In fact the term 'functional disorder' is used because the problem is not in the organ or system itself but in the way it functions.

A functional disorder is classified by the type of organ or system that it affects. IBS is part of the functional bowel disorders, with symptoms attributable to the middle or lower gastrointestinal tract.

How is the diagnosis made?

Initially IBS was an exclusion diagnosis. This means that after doctors ruled out all possible organic causes of symptoms (Crohn's disease, diverticulitis, ulcerative colitis, gastroenteritis or colon cancer) they would give patients this diagnosis. A lot of research has been done in the past twenty years that allows for a clear and reliable diagnosis to be made without having to go through the whole exclusion process, which can entail some very painful or uncomfortable investigations. In fact, a group of specialists called The Rome Group have been meeting in Rome since 1989 to study IBS and have come up with a simple way of diagnosing IBS through the symptoms (listed in the next section) that people present with. The guidelines proposed by The Rome Group are now generally regarded as the most useful way of diagnosing IBS.

Symptoms

So let's look now at something that you probably know quite a lot about: the symptoms associated with Irritable Bowel Syndrome.

According to The Rome Group's criteria, the key symptom for a reliable diagnosis of IBS is recurrent abdominal pain or discomfort for at least three days per month in the past three months (with symptom onset at least six months prior to diagnosis) associated with two or more of the following.

1 Improvement of pain or discomfort with defecation.

2 Onset associated with a change in frequency of stool.

3 Onset associated with a change in form (appearance) of stool.[1]

Other symptoms that are usually described by IBS sufferers and that support the diagnosis are:

1 Abnormal stool frequency — this could be either three or more bowel movements per day or fewer than three bowel movements per week.

2 Abnormal stool form — stool is considered abnormal when it presents in a hard/lumpy state or in a loose/watery state.

3 Abnormal stool passage — reports of straining, urgency or feelings of incomplete evacuation.

4 Passage of mucus — passage of a slimy substance by the rectum.

5 Bloating or abdominal distension — enlargement of the abdominal region.

6 Production of excessive gas.

7 Occurrence of pain and/or distension after eating.

People who suffer from IBS also have a high frequency of symptoms from the rest of the body, such as indigestion, nausea, head and back aches, fatigue, frequent urination or painful sexual intercourse, to name just a few.

Although IBS is no longer diagnosed by exclusion, and physical investigations are minimal, doctors are very alert for any of the so-called 'red flag' symptoms. Red-flag symptoms are those that a doctor would not expect to see in IBS and are usually associated with organic diseases such as Crohn's disease and ulcerative colitis. Whenever one or more of these symptoms presents, doctors will frequently order further investigations to help rule out organic disease.

You should consult your general practitioner or IBS specialist if you suffer from any of the following red-flag symptoms that we talked about earlier:

* recent unexplained weight loss

* passing blood with your stools

* fever

* being awakened by IBS-like symptoms

* a rapid and persistent unexplained change in bowel habit (if you are over 40).

Different types of IBS

For greater ease in differentiating patients when it comes to treatment approaches or research, The Rome Group came up with four different types of IBS presentations. Which of the following seems more like you?

IBS-D: This is the sub-type in which diarrhoea is predominant. Most of the bowel movements consist of loose or watery stools. IBS-D is often associated with a higher rate of urgency to go to the toilet.

IBS-C: This is the sub-type in which constipation is predominant. Most bowel movements consist of hard, lumpy stools. Straining on the toilet is very common in IBS-C.

IBS-M: This is a mixed sub-type in which diarrhoea and constipation alternate.

IBS-U: This form of IBS is not categorised into a sub-type due to a lack of abnormality in stool consistency to meet the criteria of any of the other sub-types.

Explaining symptoms

As we have seen, the two main diagnostic criteria for IBS relate to abdominal pain and to the frequency and consistency of stools. Researchers have found that altered patterns of motility and increased sensitivity in the bowel are the best explanation for these key symptoms. Let's have a closer look at what is happening and how it relates to your symptoms.

Motility

Several researchers have found that the motility — speed of movement — in the muscles of the bowel of IBS patients is different from the motility in healthy people or people with similar symptoms to IBS but who are suffering from an organic disease. A recent review of studies[2] showed that in patients with diarrhoea-predominant IBS, there seems to be an increase in contractions of the muscle, which results in the stool passing through the bowel more quickly. They also note that a decrease in these contractions seems to happen in patients with constipation-predominant IBS.

But how does the speed of contractions relate to the symptoms of constipation or diarrhoea? If your stools move through your bowel too quickly, the intestine will not have time to absorb as much water as it could, so your stool will be more watery when it reaches the end of the colon, hence diarrhoea. If they take too long to move then your intestine will continue to absorb water, which will dry up the stools and make them even harder to move, hence constipation. Also, frequent movement or spasms can cause pain, as well as trapped faeces or gas due to reduced bowel movement.

Bowel sensitivity

IBS patients seem to have a heightened sensitivity to the stretching of the bowel when stools or gas are passing, which leads to pain or feelings of discomfort such as bloating. Several researchers have shown that people with IBS are more sensitive to pain in their bowels and experience more pain when their bowels move than people who don't have IBS.

What causes IBS?

Although it has been a greatly studied subject, especially in the past twenty years, specialists have not yet found a single cause that explains IBS. They have found, though, that both biological and psychological factors seem to contribute to the trigger, aggravation and maintenance of symptoms.

The best explanation that scientists have come up with so far is that there seems to be a problem in the communication between the brain and the gut. In the gut we have many nerves that not only transmit messages to the brain about what is happening in the gut (for example, pain), but they also receive messages from the brain that influence the working of the gut (for example, an urge to go to the toilet if the body feels stress). These are very normal processes and in most people they don't cause any trouble. In IBS, however, it seems that the transmission of these messages between brain and gut gets amplified and twisted. The brain receives more messages from the gut than usual and the gut responds to messages from the brain more easily. It is as if the communication is always overworking. It is also thought that this disruption of communication between brain and gut can be triggered by biological, social or psychological sources, which we will review next.

Triggers of IBS

Triggers are not causes of IBS, rather they are factors that seem to be associated with the onset, exacerbation or maintenance of IBS symptoms, and they seem to interact with each other through the brain–gut connection. Usually these are stimuli that don't bother most people but that have an impact on people with IBS. See if any of the following examples is a trigger for you.

Food

Many people with IBS report that their symptoms get worse after they eat particular foods. Certain foods have even been dubbed as problematic in general for IBS sufferers, such as chocolate, milk, alcohol and fizzy drinks. Food allergy (an immune reaction) is very rare; what is most commonly seen is an uncomfortable reaction to certain foods, called food intolerance. Food intolerance, however, seems to be related to emotional reactions because it tends to come and go according to how a patient feels. Also, the gut seems to react to large quantities of food, so a large meal can trigger the symptoms by overexciting the sensitive nerves of the gut.

Hormones and neurotransmitters

It is thought that hormones and neurotransmitters play an important part in IBS due to their influence in the transmission of information between brain and gut. One example of this comes from stress. During periods of stress, many hormones and neurotransmitters are released by our brain, and stress has a great impact on the way our gut functions. Another example comes from menstrual cycles. In women, symptoms of IBS seem to worsen around their menstrual period, a period in which hormones go through a great change.

Infection

Although IBS is not caused by an infection, recent findings[3] show that in about 15 per cent of IBS patients, symptoms begin to show within six months of having a bout of gastroenteritis (a gastrointestinal infection that causes vomiting and diarrhoea). It is thought that the infection might make people more sensitive to, or even trigger, IBS symptoms. Another possible explanation is that the antibiotics used to clear this or other infections might kill 'good bacteria' in the gut, provoking difficulties in the digestion of certain foods, which can contribute to some symptoms. Also it has been shown that high levels of stress or emotional difficulties during a bout of gastroenteritis seem to make some people more likely to develop IBS after these infections.

Stress

You might have seen a trend in the previous triggers: that they are often associated with some form of stress. Do your symptoms seem to come along or worsen during periods of distress? It seems that in people who suffer from IBS, their gut is particularly sensitive to everyday stress (such as paying the bills, going to work). Also, people with IBS seem to react with more distress to what is happening in their gut more strongly. At times it can seem like a double-edged sword: you might experience a stressful event; your gut reacts to it, causing IBS symptoms; you become distressed about your IBS symptoms on top of the previous distress, and this amplifies or maintains your symptoms.

Knowing the basics helps but ...

At the beginning of this chapter we asked you to rate your distress related to IBS. We would like you to do it again now that you have all this information. Do you notice any change? If you are like most people you might feel a bit more empowered now that you know more about what is happening within you, or you might feel reassured that some of the things you already knew were similar to what we have presented here — but has this information altered the level of distress that IBS causes in your life? Probably not!

Information is powerful, but in a chronic illness such as IBS we might have to focus less on what we know about the illness and a bit more on what we know about ourselves.

The next two chapters will explore how your personal experience of IBS is much bigger than its symptoms, and how much dealing with IBS has cost you.

CHAPTER 2

Psychological stressors and IBS

In the previous chapter we looked at some basic information about IBS: what it is, the symptoms, how these could be understood and what triggers them. But IBS is so much more than the symptoms, and in this chapter we will reflect on some of the experiences you have had with IBS.

We would like to introduce you to Angela, who also suffers from IBS, who will keep us company throughout this book. Angela is a 22-year-old student who has been struggling with IBS for two years. The first time she encountered IBS was during a university lecture. On the way to her class she felt some discomfort and rumbles in her stomach but thought nothing of it. While in the lecture she had a sudden urge to go to the toilet for a bowel movement. She was feeling slightly nauseous, she had some abdominal pain and she started to worry that she wouldn't make it to the end of the lecture. On the other hand she was thinking of how embarrassed she would feel to have to get up during the lecture and have everyone look at her as she left. This made her very anxious and her pain increased. She eventually thought that she could not hold it any longer and got up to go to the toilet. She wasn't able to return to the lecture; she felt humiliated and was sure that everyone was wondering why she had left. She didn't think she could answer that question without feeling embarrassed.

Her symptoms increased over the following weeks, especially the pain. She would get bouts of diarrhoea and constipation with a lot of pain. Every time she would go to a lecture she would remember her first episode and feel an increase in her symptoms. Angela also noticed that situations in which she felt embarrassed would remind her of the episode and she would be unwell shortly after. She eventually gave up her degree, which was very upsetting for her. Since then, whenever she experiences symptoms she can't help but feel sad about giving up her degree because of IBS. She also feels that she has lost control of her life.

Beyond the symptoms

Have you ever just experienced a symptom? I mean really just had abdominal pain without anything going through your head, without you feeling anything? Probably not, right?

This is the result of what are some of the most important characteristics of the human being: we think, we feel and we are aware of doing so. And as an added bonus we do it all the time. Our brain is constantly giving us information about how our body is (too hot, too cold, comfortable, in pain) and how we feel (happy, anxious, sad, indifferent) as well as producing thoughts about all this information.

So it seems quite natural to say that when you are having a symptom of IBS you are probably having some thoughts and feelings about it, right? You probably experience emotions and thoughts related to your IBS even if you are not having symptoms. You might have even seen a bit of your experience in Angela's story. We've seen that Angela, for instance, would get anxious and embarrassed and she would wonder what others would think about her. What about you? What emotions or thoughts do you experience related to your IBS?

In this chapter we will focus on the feelings or thoughts that accompany symptoms of IBS, and what comes into your mind that is related to your IBS even when you are not experiencing symptoms. Basically, we would like you to look beyond the symptoms.

Emotions

First we will look at how some emotions seem to have a close connection with IBS. IBS is a particularly difficult illness to deal with, and, like Angela, a lot of people with this condition experience an overwhelming range of emotions. This is only natural; after all, some of the symptoms can be quite scary. Sometimes even more overwhelming is the situation in which the symptoms present themselves, which can be embarrassing. Feelings of sadness regarding having a condition, as well as frustration or a sense of injustice can also be hard to bear. Experiencing conflicted emotions about your IBS is therefore as common as experiencing conflicted emotions about anything else in your life.

Sometimes emotions can come out of the blue. You can find yourself feeling sad about how much IBS has taken away from your life without even experiencing the symptoms at that moment. Emotions also have a tendency to couple together, so you can feel angry about feeling anxious or feel ashamed for feeling sad.

Although we know that everyone has different emotional experiences related to IBS, we would like to present some of those most commonly reported by patients, before we move to your own personal experience.

Anxiety

This is one of the most common emotions experienced by IBS patients; it comes in many forms and is associated with many aspects of people's lives. Anxiety is connected to a feeling of fear towards a situation that might happen in the future. This is a very difficult emotion because unlike pure fear, which is a direct reaction to something threatening, anxiety will be present whether or not the threatening situation occurs. So you will experience anxiety even if what you fear might happen doesn't happen. That sounds like a very rough deal, doesn't it? Below are some examples of how anxiety might be present in IBS patients' lives.

Health anxiety

The symptoms themselves are enough to feel anxious about — after all, they are indicating that something is not right with your body, and that can be scary — but because IBS has many common traits and symptoms with more serious diseases such as colon cancer, frequently people become anxious at the possibility of IBS degenerating into something more serious in the future. Take the example of George, a 42-year-old patient with a thirteen-year history of IBS, who even after having several painful investigative procedures and being reassured by his doctor that he did not have colon cancer, would still feel great anxiety about the possibility of developing this disease.

Bowel-performance anxiety

One of the key characteristics of IBS is that people never know how their bowels are going to act (perform). This can cause anxiety in many ways, usually according to the main symptom. If diarrhoea is predominant it is common for people to be anxious about whether they are going to have access to a bathroom. Angela would feel great anxiety about whether she would feel a disabling pain when she was going to a lecture. Some people with constipation as a predominant feature will often become concerned about whether they will have a bowel movement.

Embarrassment anxiety

In general, IBS patients become extremely preoccupied with the possibility of their symptoms causing embarrassment in a public situation (something we've seen with Angela). This is a typical case of emotions becoming coupled with anxiety relating to embarrassment.

Food-related anxiety

IBS patients are usually very concerned about food, especially about how certain food products will impact their symptoms. Having a meal is compared by some to walking in a minefield where anything could set them off. This anxiety about food can become so intense that some people develop a phobia about certain foods.

While anxiety can be overwhelming and sometimes feel like it is right in your face, it is also a natural part of life. Everyone feels a bit anxious sometimes. In the case of IBS it just seems that anxiety is more connected with bowel function. This is normal because, after all, you have a bowel problem. If you had a broken foot you would probably be more anxious about falling, right? But having anxiety in itself does not mean there is something wrong with you, it is just one of those experiences that your brain is registering because you are human.

Shame and embarrassment

Like anxiety, shame and embarrassment are common emotions reported by IBS sufferers. In fact, they are sometimes associated with people feeling anxious about the possibility of embarrassing themselves.

Shame and embarrassment are often a result of the very nature of the symptoms of IBS: burping, stomach rumbles, bowel sounds, the passing of gas or soiling yourself, all of which can be frowned upon in our society. Also, any type of talk regarding bowel functions is either discouraged or used for toilet-humour jokes. It is this perception that bowel functions are associated with a lack of social manners or with immature humour that makes IBS symptoms so associated with shame and embarrassment.

Some people even feel a bit embarrassed within themselves. Take George: he would feel a deep shame for not being able to control his symptoms, but in his case he didn't care much about others' opinions, it was his own self-criticism that made him feel that way.

Angela would feel particularly ashamed for having to get up in front of her colleagues to go to the bathroom or if she had to explain why she needed to do it. This is quite common because many patients with IBS feel embarrassed trying to explain an illness that doesn't have a clear cause, and some go to the extent of saying they have an organic disease (such as Crohn's disease) to justify their behaviour to others.

Like anxiety, embarrassment and shame are natural reactions to the specific presentation of IBS, and having these feelings does not mean that you are flawed in any way.

Sadness

It is easy to understand why feelings of sadness come with IBS; after all, this illness often keeps people away from some of their favourite activities, their closest friends and family or their job. A difficulty in explaining or addressing this illness with other people promotes a sense of isolation in which patients feel misunderstood by everyone, even their doctors. Also common is a sense of grief for the loss of a particular role (such as patients who stop working because of IBS) or just for the general loss of health. Sadness tends to bring about other feelings as well: some people feel down about the embarrassment IBS causes them or feel helpless regarding their anxiety. With all this on their plate, it is no surprise that many patients also suffer from depression or from periods of lower mood.

Again we would like to stress that feeling sad about what is happening with you is a normal reaction.

Anger and frustration

For many IBS patients anger and frustration are a central part of their emotional lives. People often feel angry or frustrated with a body that seems out of control, and with other people for not understanding IBS.

Some patients find that their symptoms get worse just before or after a situation in which they felt anger. One of the most common problems following this is that many patients don't address their anger, thinking that having this emotion is wrong. They tend to bottle it up and feel even more anger or frustration in the long run.

How do you feel?

So far we have presented some of the most common emotional experiences that people with IBS report, but this book is not about other people, it is about you. We will now ask you to take some time to think about how you feel about situations in your life.

Exercise: What did I feel?

One of the best ways to stop and think about these difficult feelings that come into our lives is to write them down. In the spaces provided below we would like you to write how you felt in a particular situation that you can remember. Although we are mainly looking for those feelings associated with IBS, we encourage you to think of other situations and try to catch those same feelings in a different context — after all, having emotions is part of the whole human experience not just one particular part of it.

You can see below that we have provided you with an incomplete sentence form (I felt _____ when _____). An example of a complete sentence is: *I felt worried when I was at the shop because I felt my belly rumble.* (If you have many experiences you need to share, you can photocopy this form or use the spare ones provided in the appendix of this book.)

There are two ways you can use this exercise: you can just try to recall your experiences or you can take a couple of days to carry this book with you and register your experiences as they come along. Or you can do both. In any case, the point of this exercise is to put you in contact with your emotions both about IBS and in general. We also know that sometimes it is difficult to put emotions into words, so we have added a list of common emotional states, which we hope will help you. After you complete this exercise take a moment to simply observe the different emotions and the situations in which you experienced them.

WHAT DID I FEEL?

Examples of emotions: *I felt … angry, despaired, ashamed, anxious, frustrated, miserable, guilty, nervous, irritated, gloomy, humiliated, tense, aggressive, mournful, blameworthy, worried, disgusted.*

I felt _____ when _____

_____

I felt _____ when _____

_____

I felt _____ when _____

_____

I felt _____ when _____

_____

I felt _____ when _____

_____

I felt _____ when _____

_____

I felt _____ when _____

_____

I felt _____ when _____

_____

I felt _____ when _____

_____

I felt _____ when _____

_____

Thoughts

In this section we will look at some of the most common thoughts that cause distressing feelings to people with IBS. Sometimes thoughts and feelings are so intertwined that it is hard to tell them apart, and it is common for people to refer to their thoughts as if they were feelings. For example, if you say, 'I felt I wouldn't be able to get to the toilet on time,' you are having the thought that you will not make it in time but the feeling might actually be anxiety or worry.

It might have happened in the previous exercise that some of the underlying situations in which you felt a certain way were related to a particular thought. As you may remember, Angela would become anxious at the thought of having to explain her situation to someone else. If you think about it, this is very common. For instance, the memory of a deceased relative with whom you were very close can bring about feelings of sadness for the loss of them, or can bring happiness for the good times you both had, or even a mix of both.

As we have seen for emotions, thoughts about IBS can be very specific due to the nature of the illness. Most of them revolve around the features of the symptoms, about the consequences of symptoms or the anticipation of these symptoms. Some might be related less to the symptoms than to a general sense of something not being well.

Thoughts can take different forms, such as a picture flashing in your mind, a memory, a sentence that rings in your mind or an ongoing comment about what you are doing.

We will look at Angela's story as an example of some of the most common thoughts associated with IBS. When she has symptoms, Angela reports thoughts such as, 'I will have an accident,' 'I can't hold it any longer,' 'I'll make a spectacle of myself,' 'Everyone is looking at me.' This leads her to feel anxious and embarrassed. Regarding her pain, Angela reports thinking, 'This is unbearable,' 'I can't handle this pain, it is too much for me,' 'It will always ruin my life,' 'I can't concentrate with all this pain.' This leads her to feel helpless and sad. Even when she isn't having any symptoms Angela has thoughts popping into her mind about it, such as, 'I will not be able to go to lectures because of my IBS,' 'My life is out of control,' 'I will always be ill.'

Do any of these sound familiar?

Maybe you are more like George, who keeps thinking, 'The doctors missed something,' 'I am going to develop colon cancer because of this,' 'I hate myself for having this,' 'I am a burden to everyone around me.'

Whatever it is that goes through your mind, it is part of you and of your experience with IBS, but there are also many other thoughts that don't have to do with IBS that go through your mind, and those are a part of you too. The IBS-related thoughts probably just feel more relevant because they are associated with distressing emotions and symptoms. Later in the book we will look at how some forms of dealing with IBS experiences can actually make it worse, and how a new perspective might help.

Putting it all together

It is time now to integrate all of what we have addressed in this chapter. We have introduced you to the concept that IBS is more than symptoms; there are thoughts and feelings associated with it as well. We've explained that even though these thoughts and feelings are part of a bigger natural process (being human) they are distressing and cause a lot of pain. We have also shown you that thoughts and feelings can pop up even if you have not had an IBS symptom. And that is why before we move to the next chapter — where we will explore further the nature of suffering in IBS — we would like you to take some time and work on an exercise that might help make some sense of all this.

Exercise: Experiencing and doing

In order to gain a better sense of how symptoms, thoughts and feelings associated with IBS interact, we will ask you to keep a diary of your experiences for the next week. Use this diary to track the presentation of IBS stressors, the symptoms (if you felt any), the thoughts and the feelings that caused you distress in a particular situation and how you reacted. Try to describe the situation in a concise manner and try to describe how you behaved as a consequence of the episode.

Also see what came first in these situations and give an order to the stressors. (You will find extra copies of the form in the appendix of this book.) Try carrying this book around so that you can quickly register any experience or commit to doing it at a particular time of the day. (We have also included an example from Angela, which may help you prepare your own chart.)

IBS has many factors that contribute to stress, which then contributes to the maintenance of the illness itself, the symptoms, thoughts and feelings. Although all of these are distressing, they are also a part of the human experience. What we are going to say now might seem strange, but we think that perhaps some of the suffering in IBS might not come from having these distressing experiences, but from how people with IBS react to these experiences. We are not saying that these experiences don't contribute to the suffering, but that maybe the key lies elsewhere. We invite you to stay with this notion for a while before turning to the next chapter even though it might be a bit uncomfortable. Ready? Okay, let's see what we meant by that.

WHAT DID I EXPERIENCE? WHAT DID I DO?				
Situation	Symptoms	Feelings/ emotions	Thoughts	What did I do?

ANGELA'S DIARY				
Situation	**Symptoms**	**Feelings/ emotions**	**Thoughts**	**What did I do?**
Monday At home after breakfast.	1. Pain, diarrhoea	3. Despair, sadness	2. I can't hold it any longer! I'll soil myself!	Lay in bed after emptying my bowels.
Tuesday Friend called inviting me for coffee.	No symptoms	2. Anxiety, fear	1. What if there isn't an available toilet at the coffee shop?	Turned down my friend's invitation.
Tuesday At the shop buying cigarettes.	1. Bloating, gas	2. Shame, embarrassment	3. I'm going to embarrass myself. Everyone is looking at me and feeling disgusted.	Ran out of the store and back home as fast as I could.
Wednesday In the toilet having a bowel movement.	3. Diarrhoea	1. Anxiety	2. I should check my stools to see if everything is okay.	Spent five minutes going through my stools to make sure there wasn't any blood.
Thursday At my mum's house.	1. Pain	3. Hopelessness, anger	2. I can't bear this pain! I hate this so much!	Started shouting and fighting with my mum when she asked how I was.

CHAPTER 3

How do you cope with IBS, and at what cost?

In the first two chapters of this book we discussed the symptoms of IBS and the thoughts and emotions that directly result from the experience of having IBS, and how distressing and uncomfortable they can be. We have seen how they seem to be all interconnected and to influence each other. But still, we left you with a thought in the previous chapter that all of this might not be the core of suffering in IBS. Before we clarify what we mean by 'suffering in IBS', let's take a look at one of the most common reactions to the IBS experience. You might have come across this in the exercise at the end of Chapter 2: avoidance.

Avoiding distress — the natural solution

So far we have seen that the experience of IBS can cause a lot of distress in the people who have it. The symptoms are unpleasant, there are many uncomfortable emotions and thoughts that come attached, and this can all be overwhelming.

As human beings we long ago developed a mechanism that in most instances works very well for our survival: we avoid things that are dangerous for us or that cause us discomfort. Think of the primitive man, in the wild with all sorts of creatures that could attack and cause serious harm to him. By being able to think ahead and predict where these creatures would be, he was able to avoid places where he would be most vulnerable or unprotected, and therefore he increased his chances of survival. If the weather was cold, man learned how to avoid it by staying in caves or, later on, by building houses. We have become such experts at avoiding or controlling things that make us uncomfortable or physically vulnerable that it is probably the most common reaction people have. So we started applying the same solution for internal discomfort. For example, if we have a headache we might avoid walking around too much so that it doesn't get worse; if watching a drama makes us sad we might avoid it and watch a comedy instead; if we are having troublesome thoughts we might try not to think of it or to distract ourselves with something else. So, avoidance of distressing events is well ingrained in us. Added to this is society's reinforcement of this sense through such expressions as, 'If you can't stand the heat, get out of the kitchen' or 'Out of sight, out of mind.'

So, with the pressures of evolution and generations of a society telling us that we should avoid discomfort, it seems that avoiding is almost the natural thing to do.

The cost of avoidance

So, avoidance looks like a brilliant answer to everything, doesn't it? If something is distressing, avoid it. Sounds reasonable … or does it? The problem is that avoidance, especially avoidance of internal discomfort, usually comes with a heavy cost. Let's look at another bit of Angela's story.

As you can see from Angela's avoidance list, there were many things in life that she was keeping herself away from. After all, she was protecting herself from undesirable symptoms, feelings and thoughts. She stopped going to her lectures, meeting her friends and going on holidays, which was fine for a while … until Angela started to realise that because of all this avoidance, she had to drop her degree, which was very important to her; she hardly left the house or talked with other people unless it was in what she considered a 'safe place'. Even when she was out and talking to other people she was so focused on not getting ill, making sure that she had a toilet available or keeping herself from eating anything that could trigger her symptoms, she hardly enjoyed these outings.

Exercise: What have I been avoiding?

In the table below, try to identify distressing situations that you have been avoiding, and why. See if this avoidance is allowing you to not come into contact with unpleasant symptoms, thoughts or feelings regarding your IBS. After coming up with as many examples as you can, look at Angela's example on the following table; it might help you to come up with some more items.

What situations have I been avoiding?	Why? *I don't want to come in contact with* … (symptoms, feelings, thoughts)
1.	
2.	
3.	
4.	
5.	
6.	
7.	
8.	
9.	
10.	

ANGELA'S AVOIDANCE LIST	
What situations have I been avoiding?	**Why? *I don't want to come in contact with ... (symptoms, feelings, thoughts)***
1. Going to lectures	Pain, diarrhoea, embarrassment
2. Meeting my friends	Anxiety, thinking that I'm going to get ill
3. Exercising	Pain
4. Trying new foods	My symptoms, worrying if the new food will trigger my symptoms
5. Talking to people	Sadness, memories of what I am missing because of my IBS
6. Having a relationship	Feeling ashamed, thinking that I might be rejected
7. Going on holidays	Nervousness, worrying about where toilets will be available
8. Taking the bus	Anxiety, thinking that I might have to leave at any point, thinking I'll make a mess of myself, embarrassment
9. Going to the shops	Thinking that there might be a cue, I might have an accident
10. Explaining to my family	Anger, thinking how they don't understand me, sadness, thinking I'm all alone

This was Angela's darkest moment and the point at which her suffering was at its worst, because she realised that in order to avoid the stressful symptoms, thoughts and emotions that come with IBS she had given up things that mattered most to her. And the worst was that although this avoidance initially lessened her flare-ups, they were still occurring every now and again.

Does Angela's story sound familiar?

Have you noticed that every time you avoid a situation or an event because these might cause discomfort, you are also narrowing the options available to you? It is a trade-off, right? By avoiding, you are gaining the benefit of perhaps feeling a little bit more comfortable now, but you don't get any other benefits that could have resulted from stepping into that situation. As we saw, Angela traded her education for not feeling ashamed and anxious. Does that sound like a good deal?

By avoiding situations because they might be uncomfortable, you are narrowing your life. It is like you are building a house and you have several stacks of bricks. You can only see the bricks that sit on top of these stacks and as you look around you see that some stacks look nicer than others. On top of some stacks are nice, shiny new bricks that represent positive sensations, thoughts and feelings. Other stacks have broken, filthy bricks that represent IBS symptoms, thoughts and feelings. So you choose to build only with the nice bricks and avoid touching the nasty-looking ones. When you build the house with only the shiny bricks, there aren't many of them and so the house is very small and, you guessed it, narrow.

If it got you a bigger space to live in, would you be willing to build your house with some of the other bricks too?

Experiential avoidance

Avoidance can take many forms and be very tricky, so we need to be clear about what we mean by avoidance. Experiential avoidance is an unwillingness to stay in contact with painful experiences. It is very easy to understand this when we are talking about open behaviours such as not going to a certain place, or running away from a situation, but avoidance can also occur in more subtle ways. If you think about it, every time you try to do something to change a thought or feeling about your IBS you are actually avoiding the experience of IBS. Things such as trying to distract yourself, or trying to think happy thoughts in times when you are having IBS-related thoughts or feelings is a way of avoiding the experience. Another example is continual visits to the doctor to seek reassurance that your situation is normal and that it has not evolved into something more serious — this can be viewed as an attempt to avoid distressing thoughts or feelings related to your symptoms being more serious or dangerous to your health.

What research into Acceptance and Commitment Therapy (ACT) has proven so far is that these types of avoidances do not work — in fact, they make things worse and cause more suffering.[1]

Suffering and IBS

IBS is tricky: it brings with it distress, and distressing situations also seem to make it worse. It is a catch-22 condition, in which the main advice is 'Don't feel stressed!' And you try your best not to. You avoid situations in which distressing symptoms, thoughts or feelings might occur so that you can have some control over the illness, but then the flipside of the coin hits you. You begin to associate the symptoms with the situations in which these may occur. You start avoiding those situations in order to avoid symptoms, thoughts and feelings. The things you had planned for your life start to be put on hold. A sense of loss of vitality starts to creep in. You don't do what you used to. Your goals start to change because getting close to them would imply coming into contact with IBS experiences. You start to yearn for the life you wanted to live but that you are not living right now. And guess what comes with that suffering: more distress.

Take a moment to think … does this sound familiar?

One of the most common complaints about IBS is not really about the symptoms, but about how dealing with IBS has changed people's lives. Many patients report feeling trapped by their symptoms. They stop participating in activities that they valued in order to gain some control over the disease, and later they find that missing out on those activities is actually more emotionally painful than the disease itself. Angela felt the worst in her life when she realised how much she had traded for some peace of mind and more physical comfort.

We know IBS is painful and can cause stress and other emotions, though we ask you which is more painful: having IBS or not living your life?

Researchers have come across this question many times when studying the quality of life of IBS patients.[2] Quality of life is composed of many domains of life. Health plays a major part in quality of life, but so do job satisfaction, the ability to perform daily activities and time for leisure or socialising, just to name a few. What researchers found was that IBS patients who tried to reduce their symptoms by avoiding situations that caused distress and/or led to flare-ups did not have any better quality of life than other patients. In fact, the more patients avoided their condition the worse their quality of life seemed to be. We think this happens because all the effort that patients go through to avoid their IBS experience ends up interfering with other domains in life. So by trying only to address their health quality of life, most patients end up reducing their chances to have a better quality of life in other domains.

So, it is clear that much IBS suffering occurs because the things you do to avoid undesired IBS experiences also prevent you from doing what you value in life.

The trades of life

Before we examine your experience of suffering and where avoidance is costing you quality of life, we would like to give you some examples of common areas where people with IBS usually make this trade-off.

Work

Stopping work altogether, reducing hours or taking a job that you don't really want just because it allows you to avoid more stressful situations are all examples of actions people with IBS take that in the long run increase their suffering by keeping them away from professional goals.

Leisure activities

Many patients avoid them and suffer because they no longer get the enjoyment from these activities.

Exercise

Avoiding exercise can be difficult if you used to be an active person, and it can also bring problems such as a lack of fitness, poorer health or reduced social contact.

Daily activities

Going to the shops, picking up the kids from school and paying bills are situations commonly avoided that could have both practical as well as emotional suffering attached to them when avoided.

Travelling/holidays

Travel is one of the worst nightmares for IBS patients. The buses, trains, planes: 'Will a toilet be available?' 'Everything will be unknown where I'm going.' It is easy to avoid. But what about your desire to be able to move freely and maybe explore new places? Does it hurt not to answer that call?

Social interactions

Family, friends, co-workers — they can all be a source of stress; they can also be very supportive and understanding. Avoiding them only brings further isolation.

Food

Being constantly on the lookout to see if a food will bring you harm; not allowing yourself to enjoy new flavours; reducing your source of nutrients — avoidance of food can not only make life a bit blander, it can also come with a health price when some essential food products are avoided.

Seeking reassurance

It is common for people to put their whole life on hold worrying about their diagnosis and the evolution of the disease. All the time spent at the doctor's and all the painful examinations are more ways of getting away from the scary thought, 'They must have missed something serious.'

These examples are just a sample of areas in which important aspects of your quality of life might be traded in attempts to experience less IBS-related discomfort.

Exercise: What is avoidance costing you?

This is a more elaborate version of the avoidance exercise, and you can take some of the situations you wrote down for that exercise to help you with this one. Here we would like you to think about how you try to avoid, control or change distressing situations related to your IBS. After this we would like you to consider if your symptoms, thoughts or feelings increase or decrease by avoiding a certain situation, both in the short and long term. Finally we would like you to reflect on the impact of avoidance strategies on your quality of life, and what you are giving up.

Don't forget that we are looking for the situations in which you are unwilling to stay in contact with your IBS experiences. These could even include situations such as watching TV or sleeping all day to avoid thinking about your symptoms, or taking drugs or drinking too much alcohol. As we have seen, avoidance can take many forms.

In the following chart, list situations in which you have avoided aspects of your IBS. (You will find more copies of this form in the appendix at the end of the book if you need them.) Take a look at Angela's example on the next page if you feel a bit stuck.

How do you cope with IBS, and at what cost?

Situation	Experience avoided (symptom, thought, feeling)	Short-term effect	Long-term effect	Long-term effect on quality of life

ANGELA'S COSTS OF AVOIDANCE

Situation	Experience avoided (symptom, thought, feeling)	Short-term effect	Long-term effect	Long-term effect on quality of life
Did not go to lectures	Thoughts of being ill, feeling embarrassed	Some relief	None	Gave up my degree.
Cancelled meetings with my friends	Anxiety about whether a toilet would be available, symptoms	Some relief	None	My friends and I are not as close anymore.
Carry my medication everywhere	Symptoms, feeling helpless or out of control	Complete relief	None	I am always wondering if I have my pills, and this interferes with my concentration.
Not approaching men	Feelings of rejection, shame, thinking I am not worthy	None	None	Haven't had a relationship in three years.
Stopped eating certain foods that might be related to my symptoms	Symptoms	Works sometimes	None	I still have my symptoms no matter how careful I am with my diet.

Stopped exercising	Symptoms, mainly pain	Some relief	None	My doctor told me that my blood pressure is too high because of my lack of exercise.
Drinking to numb myself on certain days	Symptoms, sadness, hopelessness, thinking that my life is ruined and that I will never get better	No relief	None	Always end up being sick, feeling sorry for myself for doing something so stupid and thinking that I probably just made things worse.
Trying every new medication	Symptoms	Some relief	None	New medication works for a while and then the symptoms come back.

If you are anything like Angela or like many IBS patients, going through this exercise might have been very difficult. It is quite hard sometimes to see in black and white, in your own words and based on your own experience, that all those efforts to make yourself better are actually not having any effect — or very limited effect — on your condition. And even harder is noticing that acting in that way has kept you away from the life you want.

Like we said before, while we see that IBS is difficult, we don't believe that it is the experience of IBS that keeps you from enjoying life, but the way you respond to it. We believe that most people with IBS are actually trying to escape their experiences because they want to move their lives in a certain direction that they value. What happens is that they seem to have made a deal with themselves in which they will only move forward if their IBS and all that is attached to it goes away.

Do you feel like there is a lot you want to do that you have put on hold because of your IBS?

Being in this position — in which it seems that you have tried everything — can be scary, but it can also be empowering. If what you have always done isn't working, maybe it is not because you didn't do it right or didn't try hard enough. If you are like most people with IBS you have tried very hard to control your symptoms and the stress associated with them, but perhaps this strategy is part of the problem.

While this can be hard to acknowledge, it is also worth noting that it is not *you* that isn't working right. You, as a person, are not broken and you do not need to be fixed. It is the *strategy* you are using that is the problem. Maybe it is time to try something new …

What can you do differently?

Picture a pit of quicksand. Do you have it in your mind? Now, if you were to fall into it, what would be the best course of action? You've probably seen enough Tarzan or Indiana Jones movies to know that the more you struggle and try to step out of the quicksand, the more you will sink. In fact, the best thing to do involves you coming into contact with as much quicksand as you can. To come out of the pit you have to lie on the quicksand, having as much of the surface of your body in contact with it so that your weight gets spread out. This allows you to float rather than sink. This is a very good example of how what at first seems illogical is actually the best option. The approach that we suggest in this book is very similar to this situation. Instead of trying not to have your symptoms, thoughts and feelings, we would like you to come into contact with them, so that they stop being reasons for not doing this or not doing that. Basically, we suggest that you shift your focus from controlling or getting rid of IBS to living a full life while having IBS.

We know this is a difficult thing to try. But on the other hand you have tried the controlling-symptoms way and you've seen where that has led you. If we were to give you more strategies to eliminate/control/change your symptoms/thoughts/feelings wouldn't we just be giving you more of the same?

Time to choose

Let's say that we have two gifts to give you and you have to choose one.

Gift 1: In this gift you have a pill that will reduce your experience of IBS symptoms, thoughts or feelings. But in order for the pill to take effect you will have to give up all the hopes, dreams and goals you had planned for your life once your IBS has gone.

Gift 2: In this gift, there is no pill. The symptoms, thoughts and feelings will still be there, sometimes better, sometimes worse. But in this gift there are skills that will help you to get in touch with where you want to go in life. There are also skills that will enable you to come into contact with your IBS symptoms and feelings while still moving in the direction you value. In this gift you will be taught how to step back and just notice your thoughts, taking from them the useful parts that will lead you to where you want to go in life. With this gift you will be able to truly live your life while taking IBS with you, instead of living your life in order to get rid of IBS.

Which one do you choose?

If you chose gift 1, it may be that our approach is not right for you at this point in your life. We recommend that you keep this book; it may be that at some point in the future it could be more useful to you. If more control and a reduction of symptoms is what you most want, the rest of this book may not be overly helpful. But feel free to read it anyway; you may discover something else useful in its pages. Go back over this book many times and in particular, spend time asking yourself the questions this book asks, and doing the written exercises.

If you chose gift 2, turn the page and start building the map of the directions you most value in life.

CHAPTER 4

Mapping your direction

So far most of the work we have done in this book has been about building a picture of what is going on with you. We have explored the experience of having IBS, from the symptoms to the way it makes you feel and think. We have also seen that the way people react to IBS tends to get them off track from what they really want to do in life.

Because you have been dealing with IBS for a while, it is easy to lose sight of why you wanted to get rid of the experiences of IBS in the first place. Regaining contact with what you want your life to be about is where the real work starts. In this chapter we will help you create a map of where you want your life to go. This is about figuring out how you want to live your life and not about how to live it so that IBS doesn't bother you.

What are values?

Figuring out how to live *with* IBS instead of living to try to control IBS involves spending some time focusing on values and goals. But what do we mean by values?

Values reflect what is most important to you; they bring meaning to your life. When you are living according to your values you feel more alive and have a sense of purpose and consistency.

Values are like directions on a compass that helps orientate your life. When you look at your personal compass, you may have a general idea of the direction in which you want to take your life. These directions can be almost anything. Many people describe values such as being a good friend, a good parent, a loving husband or wife, someone who gives back to the community, to name a few.

One of the most important characteristics of values is that they are personal and individual. Everyone has their own set of directions that makes them feel like a full human being. So, values are not what morality or society imposes upon you by fear or guilt, but something that you, and only you, assign importance to because they bring you a sense of vitality. Your personal compass is yours and yours alone.

Another characteristic of values is that they can never be achieved — they are only a direction, not a destination. If you think of it in compass terms again, if heading east is important to you, values will give you that direction but you can never arrive at east; you move towards east, but there is always more east to go. So, values are different from goals. On your way heading east you might create goals that you want to achieve and that are consistent with the direction you want to take. You might want to get to Russia. That is east, but from there you can go further east and set a new goal to go to Canada, and once you arrive there you can always go further east. You will never be able to say, 'I have arrived at east.' This is much like the example of having the value of being a good friend. You can never say, 'That's it! I'm a good friend, so I don't have to do anything else.' There is always something more you can do tomorrow that shows you are a good friend, or maybe the day after, and so on.

Living according to your values is not always easy. Much like the compass, you only get a rough idea of which direction you want to head in, but you don't get any information about what sort of things you are going to face by going in that direction. Let's take the example of climbing a mountain. When you start at the base of the mountain you look at it and you have an idea of the path you want to take, and you put on your hiking boots and start to climb. But suddenly some obstacles that you didn't see from the base of the mountain appear in front of you — a big rock blocking your way, or a huge pit of mud. You look up and because you are too close you can't see the mountaintop, so you grab your trusty compass that tells you that the way towards where you want to go is through that obstacle. At this point you can choose to go around and get off the track or you can stay on track and work with the obstacle, knowing that you are going in the direction you really want.

This brings us to what is probably the most important feature of values: they are choices. It is easy to find reasons not to follow a value. In the mountain metaphor, you could come up with reasons such as 'It's too hard' or 'It's too risky.' This is much like what we find in our lives. You want to be a good friend but going out to socialise is too hard. When such reasons start to orient your choices instead of your own sense of direction, you get sidetracked from your values — and this brings the pain of a life not lived.

The road to living your life like you really want to, in spite of your IBS, is long and hard. There will be difficult times, there will be great times. Either way there will be choices to be made. In this chapter we will explore what you value the most so that when confronted with these choices you can have your compass handy and may be able to choose to move in the direction of your values.

Defining your values

Now that you have a good idea of what we mean by values, it is time to take a look at what really matters to you. Because this is a difficult task we will suggest some areas (or 'domains') that seem to be common to many people. There may well be some more areas that we haven't listed that you feel are important for you. For now we will focus on: family, intimate relationships, friends, work, health and growth and learning. This doesn't mean that all people value these domains or that they value them in the same way. They are just the most common.

Exercise: Exploring your values

This exercise focuses on how you would like your life to be in seven domains, six of which we have presented before as the most common ones that people seem to give great value. You'll also see that there is an extra one without any theme to it. People value different things and some of them are quite original. This seventh domain will be your own personal domain.

Now we would like you to dig deep into your dreams and aspirations. Set aside your current predicament and think of how you would most want things to be in each domain. In each of the sections listed below, describe how you would want to experience each of the domains regardless of your age or life circumstances.

Family: Describe in a few sentences how you would like your relationship to be with your parents, children, siblings and perhaps even your extended family. If the world were perfect what would these relationships be like? What qualities would you bring to these relationships to make them the best possible?

Intimate relationships: Consider the relationship you have with that special person who is closest to you. Think about what it is in that relationship that is so valuable for you. Even if you don't have anyone you consider intimate at this moment, think about what you consider to be the most important thing in a relationship. Write down a few sentences on the qualities of an ideal intimate relationship and what this would bring to you. Think about the kind of person with whom you would most want to share that relationship.

_____

_____

_____

_____

_____

_____

_____

_____

Friendships: These types of relationships can cover a wide variety of people. You can consider how you relate to close friends, work friends or acquaintances. Write a few sentences about how relating to these people would look like in an ideal world. If you really got to choose, what kind of a friend would you be?

_____

_____

_____

_____

_____

_____

_____

_____

Work: Think about what sort of valued qualities come with having a job or volunteering. You could think of a personal endeavour, like a career, that you might have given up on or seen being affected by your IBS. What type of work would make the most use of your special set of skills? What would a job that gives you meaning look like? What would be the qualities of such a perfect job or volunteer position?

_____

_____

_____

_____

_____

_____

_____

Health: Think about the importance of keeping healthy. Do exercising, eating right and having a good night's sleep play an important role in your life? Write down a few sentences about how you would like to take care of your body in ideal circumstances.

_____

_____

_____

_____

_____

_____

_____

_____

_____

Growth and learning: Think about how important it is for you to learn new skills or gain knowledge. Is improving yourself something that drives you? Write down the qualities related to your personal growth as a human being that you would like to develop throughout your life, regardless of any difficult circumstances or age. If you could choose to make your life be about your own growth and learning, what would that life look like? What would you do differently?

_____

_____

_____

_____

_____

_____

Your own personal value: Think about something that has not been listed before but that is really important to you. Some examples could be issues of spirituality or having a hobby; for other people community participation or citizenship is important. Write a few sentences about something you feel truly passionate about, what it brings to you and how it would look like in an ideal world.

_____

_____

_____

_____

_____

_____

_____

Defining your values can be a hard task. We know that as you worked through this exercise your mind may have been telling you things like, 'It's impossible, I can't do that, what's the point in thinking about how I want it to be, my IBS will stop me from getting a life like that.' We understand this and we will help you with it in other chapters. For now, we ask you to let those kinds of thoughts be there and still keep on thinking about how you would most want your life to be, if you really could choose.

Being able to put into words what you want your life to be about is a good first step, but it doesn't give you the full flavour of what it would look like to live that full life. That is why we are going to persist in the exploration of values with an exercise that people find helpful to get in touch with that feeling of what it is like to live a fulfilling life.

Exercise: Your 100th birthday

Take a minute to close your eyes and imagine that you have just celebrated your 100th birthday. You have lived a fulfilling life and made it to this astonishing age. There is a big celebration and everyone you care about is there. Because this is an imagination exercise we do mean *everyone* you care about is there: family, friends, people you admire, even people who are no longer living but who hold a special place in your heart. Imagine where the party is being held, how the room looks, if it is a special place for you. Think of what sort of music will be playing and even what sort of aromas you can smell from the food being served.

As a special birthday treat you have asked someone in particular to say a few words about your life. Think about someone you would like to speak on your behalf about the amazing life you led. Jot that person's name down below.

Speaker: _____

Now imagine what you most want this person to say about you and your life, regardless of what you think they might actually say. Remember you have lived a full life, so this person is describing the 'you' that lived according to your values, not the 'you' that is currently in a difficult situation. Try not to let the reality of now interfere with the description of this ideal future 'you'. Imagine the speech this person is making, and write down what you think this person would say about your ideal 'you' and the life you led.

Now take a moment to reflect on what you heard in this speech. What does this tell you about your values — about what really matters to you, deep in your heart? Were there any particular domains that stood out in the speech? Maybe some themes such as family, relationships, friends, work, health or growth that we explored in the previous exercise came up. Or maybe another domain that is very relevant to you. It is fine if you noticed that you value some areas more than others — after all, we are all different. Re-read what you just wrote and jot down the values you can find in it.

_____

_____

_____

_____

In this exercise it is easy to see how important values are; how present they are in our lives and how much they guide us. But this exercise doesn't have to be a 'once-only affair'. Why not try choosing someone else to give the speech? What if you could have yourself giving the speech? See what happens.

Living values and goals

We hope the previous exercises have given you a good idea of what really matters to you and the directions in which you would like to take your life. This is essential, because now you can start to be a bit more specific and begin to look at the goals that are consistent with your values.

Like values, goals orient you in a direction, but they have an end point and an outcome that you can achieve. So, goals are like points on a map that you can arrive at on your way east. They are achievable and therefore very important because they give you a more concrete sense of movement. Having a values-consistent goal is also essential to move in your desired direction because it will allow you to plan the actions you have to take to get there.

Before you start the next exercise we need to offer a brief note of warning about some goals that are impossible to achieve — we call these 'dead-man goals'.

Dead-man goals are very tricky and they can easily creep into the goals you would like to define. Examples of dead-man goals include, 'I would like to never feel pain again,' 'I would like to never feel embarrassed again,' 'I would like to never feel distressed about my IBS again.' We call these dead-man goals because to achieve them, you would have to be dead. Whenever a goal involves removing a human experience such as physical sensations, thoughts or feelings, it is quite likely that it is a dead-man goal.

Exercise: Values-consistent goals

Now let's give values-consistent goals a nice shape. Go back to your values assessments and see what stands out in each of them. What do you value in each domain? Maybe it is a closer relationship with your children or parents; maybe you would like to be a more caring partner; maybe it is being a member of a group of friends; perhaps improve your working skills; being someone who keeps fit; maybe you have a desire to learn something new every day.

For each of the value domains, try to come up with one or two specific actions that you could do that will show you that you are living that value.

Look at Angela's values and goals sheet if you need some help.

Family goals:

_____

_____

_____

Intimate-relationships goals:

_____

_____

_____

Friendships goals:

_____
_____
_____
_____

Work goals:

_____
_____
_____
_____

Health goals:

_____
_____
_____
_____

Growth and learning goals:

_____
_____
_____
_____

Your personal value goals:

_____
_____
_____
_____

ANGELA'S VALUES AND GOALS

Family
Value: I would like to be a caring daughter.
Goals: 1. Visit my parents every other month.
2. Phone them every week to let them know how I am.

Intimate relationships
Value: I would like to be in a loving relationship.
Goals: 1. Join an internet dating site.
2. Go on a date.

Friendships
Value: I would like to be there for my friend.
Goals: 1. Phone my friend to see how she is doing.
2. Go on a night out with my group of friends.

Work
Value: I would like to have a job in which I feel part of a team.
Goals: 1. Speak to a recruiter about getting back into work.
2. See what opportunities might be available and apply for a job.
3. Get to know my co-workers' names and interests.

Health
Value: I want to take care of my body and feel fit.
Goals: 1. Join my local gym.
2. Eat five portions of vegetables or fruit a day.
3. Drink 1.5 litres of water a day.

Growth and learning

Value: I would like to learn throughout my life.

Goals: 1. Finish my degree.

2. Apply for jobs that will allow my continuing development.

Personal value

Value: I would like to be more involved with the community I live in.

Goals: 1. Look for local community groups.

2. Volunteer for an activity.

Barriers

Thinking about what you value and what sorts of goals are consistent with those values is a very important first step, but this doesn't make behaving according to your values any easier. And IBS can be a pretty big barrier in the way of living according to your values.

As we have said before, IBS can produce uncomfortable experiences that can be seen as barriers on your way to living the life you want. Like in the mountain example, they can be big rocks that stand in your path up the mountain. But often how you react to these barriers is actually what dictates whether or not you follow your values.

We can say that barriers are 'clean' when, for example, you experience your distressing symptoms, thoughts or feelings about IBS and you still keep moving towards a valued direction. Take a few moments to think and jot down some situations in which you had something that you considered very important to do and you kept doing it even with IBS experiences.

_____

_____

_____

How did you feel? Probably quite good, because you were able to complete something that made you feel you had more purpose in your life.

But there are also 'dirty' barriers; the problem is that they look exactly like the clean ones. They are your symptoms, your thoughts and your feelings about IBS, but this time you let them keep you away from what you really want to do in life. Instead of going over or around the rock, you try all sorts of things to make the rock go away, or you back up the trail to try to find a new trail, or you simply stop trying to climb the mountain. Can you think of situations when IBS symptoms, thoughts or feelings kept you away from what you most valued? Write them down.

_____

_____

_____

_____

_____

IBS experiences are not the only barriers in your life. You probably can come up with time barriers or energy barriers, or barriers that are other people's expectations of you or your expectations of yourself. These often come in the form of, 'I shouldn't,' or 'I couldn't do that.' Barriers will show up in many shapes or forms but they only become clean or dirty according to the way you react to them.

In the previous chapter you saw how much avoidance of your IBS experience has cost you in quality of life. It is time now to look at how much it has driven you away from your values.

Exercise: Zorg the alien

We would like you to meet Zorg. He is an alien from a faraway galaxy who is travelling the universe to explore other life forms. In his travels Zorg has met humans before and he knows that these amazing creatures that live on Earth have these things called values that guide the way they go through life. On this visit Zorg has chosen you as his subject of study. He is up in space in his ship with a huge telescope looking down on you and just observing.

Let's suppose that Zorg had seen your values and goals list. He knows what you value and how you would behave according to those values.

For his study, and only relying on observation, Zorg has to score how much he thinks you are living your values. Remember he can only see how you act, not how you wish to act.

Based on this, how do you think Zorg would score you in the seven life domains we have talked about before? Let's say his scale goes from 0 to 10, with 0 being 'Not acting at all according to values' and 10 being 'Acting fully according to values'. What score do you think Zorg would give you?

Also think about what score you would like Zorg to give you.

How much is _____ (your name) living according to their values?

Domains	Zorg's score	Your ideal score
Family		
Intimate relationships		
Friendships		
Work		
Health		
Growth and learning		
Your personal value		

Check Zorg's scores for Angela a couple of years ago. How much is Angela living according to her values?

Domains	Zorg's score	Angela's ideal score
Family	4	8
Intimate relationships	1	9
Friendships	5	10
Work	1	9
Health	3	7
Growth and learning	4	10
Personal value	4	7

If you are anything like Angela you will see a discrepancy in how much you would like to be living according to your values and how much you are actually behaving in a way consistent with them. This allowed Angela to see what dirty barriers she was creating, and she began to take action to bring her behaviours more in line with her values. If you realised that IBS has driven you away from your values and you keep running into dirty barriers, we will help you find a way forward. This is what this book is all about: living your life like you want it to be lived rather than living according to your barriers.

In the next chapters we will help you take an alternative approach to the obstacles that life throws at you. We will encourage you to accept your IBS symptoms and the thoughts and feelings that go with these, as well as persisting in behaviours that lead you towards your values, or reducing behaviours that lead you away from your values. The work you have just done regarding your values will guide the way. As your exploration of your values continues and deepens, you may find yourself revisiting the values question over and over again: If I got to choose, what would I really want to be about?

CHAPTER 5

When to use your mind, when to lose your mind

In the previous chapters we looked at avoidance and how it can be a problem. Based on your own experience you have probably seen that in your efforts to avoid your IBS experiences (symptoms, thoughts, feelings) you have been driven away from your values, and this has caused you a lot of suffering. In this chapter we will see how our minds can interfere in how we relate to our experiences and influence our choice of avoidance over other possible behaviours.

What are minds good at doing?

When we say that our minds can be related to our suffering, this might be a bit difficult to accept. After all, over the years the human mind has allowed us to achieve great things: get to the top of the food chain, put a man on the moon, gain an understanding of the world, communicate with each other and perform quite complex tasks. All of this evolved from the mind's initial purpose, around 100,000 years ago: to protect us from harm.

To do just that, our minds are constantly categorising, judging, comparing, predicting, relating, evaluating and explaining. In other words they are continuously generating an enormous number of thoughts, feelings, rules, judgements and worries. But how aware of this are we?

Catching your thoughts

Thoughts are your mind's way of interpreting the world, and they are being generated all the time. But are you really aware of this? You would be amazed how much time can pass without us even realising that we are having thoughts. It is like having a pair of gloves that feel so natural that most of the time you don't even notice that you are wearing them. Right now we would like you to get in touch with your thoughts, to notice that they are probably occurring right here, right now while you read this book.

What are you thinking now? Take a couple of minutes to write what is going through your mind as you read this book. Jot your thoughts down as they come to you.

_____

_____

_____

_____

_____

How was that for you? Did you manage to describe many thoughts? Did you find that some thoughts led to other thoughts? Was it difficult to get everything? Were they coming to you in the form of images or sentences? Did they seem big or small? Were they coming quickly or slowly? Did you notice that even if you were thinking something like, 'I'm writing my thoughts' or 'I'm not thinking anything' these are actually thoughts?

Chances are that the space provided above was not enough to write down everything that was going on in your mind. Consider this. For a brief moment in which you paid attention to your thoughts you probably had quite a lot of them, and maybe you couldn't even attend to all the thoughts you were having. Now imagine how many thoughts you would have in an hour, a day, a month or a year. Try to remember how many times you were actually as aware of the process of thinking as you were just now with this exercise. You probably just realised that even though you are thinking all the time, you are rarely aware of the process of thinking. This exercise is just one of the many ways that we can see how much impact our mind has in our life while we are not aware of it.

Producing thoughts constantly is one of the things that the mind is really good at, as you just saw. Another great achievement of our minds is our capacity to relate between thoughts so that we can predict, categorise, compare and complete an endless number of tasks. This allows us to predict the outcomes of situations without even having to experience them directly (for example, you don't have to put your hand on a hot stove to know that it will burn you). And our minds are so good at this rule-making business that sometimes we don't even realise that we are creating rules.

Let's take a look at an example of this.

Exercise: Addition without subtraction

The mind essentially works like a big computer that keeps adding information over and over. This is very helpful because it gives us a sense of history, we can remember things from the past, we can learn new things and we can even use this new knowledge to predict what will happen in the future and practise the way we will act in case a certain event occurs. This is all done through a very complicated network of events in our brain and is facilitated by what is probably our biggest achievement as a species: language.

Let's test this theory. Suppose that we said to you that we have $1 million to give away and that all you have to do to win the million is to remember three numbers. At some point in the future (we won't tell you when) we will call you on the phone and say, 'What are the numbers?' and if you answer correctly we will give you a million dollars. The numbers we want you to remember are: 1, 2, 3. Do you have them? Good! It is very important that you don't forget them; after all, they are worth a million dollars!

So, what are the numbers again?

□ □ □

(write them here)

You probably remembered the numbers quite easily, right? Now, if we were really going to give you a million dollars (yes, we lied) wouldn't it be reasonable that you would probably remember these numbers for a long time? In fact, even knowing that we are not going to give you a million dollars, you would probably be able to recall the numbers if we saw you on the street in the next few days and asked you, 'What are the numbers?'

How about a year from now? Is it even possible that if we were to show you a suitcase full of money in a year from now and say, 'What are the numbers?' you might just remember?

Is it possible that even ten years from now, you could remember?

Have you noticed that just by reading this exercise you may well carry those numbers in your head for the rest of your life? This is how our brains work; just by raising a possible future situation you have now made a rule that if someone asks you, 'What are the numbers?' you will most likely think, '1, 2, 3' and maybe even answer that out loud. So the experience of reading this exercise has not only programmed you to think '1, 2, 3' but it could have actually programmed you to say '1, 2, 3'.

But how deep is this programming?

What if we told you that it is very important that when we ask you the question 'What are the numbers?' you *don't* think of 1, 2, 3? Let's try it.

What are the numbers?

☐ ☐ ☐

Maybe you answered 4, 5, 6 or something else that has nothing to do with 1, 2, 3. But why did you answer that? How did you know that your answer was correct? Probably because while writing it you thought, 'I have to come up with something different from 1, 2, 3.' But that reasoning itself made you think of 1, 2, 3 — and we asked you not to think about 1, 2, 3.

Isn't this amazing?

But what about things that we don't deliberately program? Let's look at another example.

Exercise: Mary, Mary, Mary

Complete the following sentences with whatever comes into your mind.

Mary had a little _____
Eeny, Meeny, Miny, _____
There's no place like _____

Did your sentences end with 'lamb', 'Moe' and 'home'? Why do you think you wrote what you wrote? Isn't it because it is part of your history?

And if you think about it, when was the last time you heard those nursery rhymes, or saw *The Wizard of Oz*?

Do you see how much programming is happening all the time? How much our actions are influenced by what is going on in our minds?

These are relatively harmless examples. But what if our minds play as much the part of the villain as the hero?

Minds — the good, the bad and the villain

As we have just seen, our minds are amazing things. They are constantly buzzing with thoughts, interpreting reality, relating everything to everything, and creating models that try to predict what is going to happen. And we listen to our minds a lot, whether consciously or not. As we said, this is very important most of the time, and sometimes even vital. For example, it is important that our minds can predict that crossing a busy street in rush hour would probably lead to being hit by a vehicle and that our minds instead orient our behaviour to go to the nearest crossing and wait for the green light. It is also important that our minds help us solve problems like how to fill in our tax return, build a bookshelf, write a shopping list and figure out which is the cheapest deal for car insurance. But what if our minds and the way they work are not always helpful? What if in the case of IBS they are actually a bit disruptive?

What if the mind is like a tool? What if the mind were like a hammer — pretty useful for some kinds of problems, such as hammering in nails or banging things into place. But what if your hammer mind is faced with a problem that is not a nail? What if IBS is more like a screw? Then maybe all the great advantages that a mind gives you are not relevant to solve this problem.

In the next part of this chapter we will look at how much listening to our minds and using our mind tool to try to solve the IBS problem can actually get in the way of acting according to what we value, and therefore bring more suffering.

Cognitive fusion

Cognitive fusion has to do with a tendency that we humans have to get caught up with the content of our thoughts. When we get fused, we take thoughts to be facts. We don't even see them as thoughts but as truths about our experience; in essence we 'buy' thoughts.

We can probably all remember times in which we jumped to a conclusion based on what we were thinking. Take for example the case of meeting one of your friends when they are in a really bad mood. One thought that can pop to mind is, 'What have I done to make them so angry?' If you buy into this thought, it is likely that you might try your best to come up with reasons why you have upset your friend and how to fix the situation. In this case you are actually interacting with your thoughts rather than with your friend. Later on you might actually find out that your friend was just having a bad day and that it wasn't at all about you.

The problem with cognitive fusion occurs when we let our thoughts dictate our actions. This happens, for example, when you have a thought such as, 'I'm not going to be able to get to a toilet; I'm going to have an accident', and that leads you to avoid a certain situation. When you have this thought you feel that an accident is probably about to occur. Memories of accidents that happened in the past or times you thought you had a near miss are likely to come up in your mind. You might start experiencing anxiety related to thoughts of being embarrassed in public if you really have an accident. When all this content comes up from one single thought and it directs your actions, we can say that you are 'buying' into that thought rather than just recognising it for what it is — a thought. We usually say that when people are fused with their thoughts, they are looking *from* their thoughts rather than looking *at* their thoughts. Your thoughts are like a pair of blue-lens sunglasses you forgot you had on: they present the world to you in this shade of blue, and you start interacting with the world as if it really was blue.

This type of cognitive fusion, in which a thought substitutes direct contact with the events happening in the present, is very common in IBS. People tend to not notice that they are interacting with thoughts rather than with the real thing. Past events are brought to the present as if they were occurring here and now. Like Ursula, who had an episode of faecal incontinence in a shop and now avoids going to shops because it reminds her of that episode and the embarrassment she felt. Also, feared future events can become present, like Angela who would not go to classes because she feared that everyone would look at her.

In these examples, we can see that Ursula and Angela were faced with a choice to act according to their values in the present moment, and yet their behaviour was dictated by their interactions with thoughts about the past and the future. It is like the focus of the mind shifts from a present with several possibilities, to a past or a future in which avoidance is the only answer.

> **Right now as you read this book, try to notice if there are particular memories of past events or predictions about the future that you get caught up in. We will return to this later.**

I am

A particularly painful form of cognitive fusion comes from the statements your mind produces about yourself — the 'I am ...' type of thoughts.

Take a few minutes to think about how you would complete the following sentences in this present moment living with your IBS.

I am _____

I am _____

I am _____

I am _____

I am _____

Whether or not you wrote them, maybe some statements like, 'I am suffering from IBS,' 'I am tired of all this pain,' 'I am losing control' might have been buzzing in the back of your mind. These types of statements are very common for people who live with IBS. When you 'buy' these types of statements you are seeing the world through the IBS glasses, rather than seeing the glasses as they are.

You could have written, 'I am a person with blue eyes,' 'I am capable of breathing,' 'I am a kind person' or 'I am reading.' All of these could be true and represent you at this moment, but when you make contact with those difficult statements about yourself, it is difficult to see the multitude of you. It's like the painful definitions that you have about yourself take over from all the other ones.

> **Right now as you read this book, try to notice if there are particular painful 'I am ...' thoughts that you get caught up in. We will return to this later.**

Evaluations

Fusing with the evaluations we make about our experiences can be particularly problematic because they can influence the way we behave. We constantly produce evaluations about our experiences, such as, 'This is good,' 'That is bad,' 'This is unbearable.' This gives situations a general positive or negative quality and guides whether we should move towards or away from such a situation. The tricky bit is that our minds also evaluate our internal experiences such as our bodily sensations, our thoughts or our emotions. All of a sudden our experiences get amplified by this quality of goodness or badness and become something that we either want to get close to or avoid.

Let's take the example of Angela again. When she had her first bout of IBS, she had all sorts of experiences going on at the same time. She was nauseous, in pain and physically uncomfortable. She was feeling anxious and embarrassed. She was thinking about what other people would say or think about her. While she was having all these experiences that she later described she was also producing several evaluations about them. Her physical symptoms were 'unbearable', her feelings 'unacceptable' and her thoughts 'crazy'. She also produced evaluations about herself as being 'broken' or 'out of control'. Although the experience had been quite unpleasant, it was amplified by the evaluations that Angela produced about it. By fusing with these evaluations she was not able to return to class because she wanted to keep those experiences as far away as possible.

> Right now as you read this book, try to notice if there are particular thoughts or emotions that you have evaluated as bad, negative, unpleasant or unbearable and that you want to keep away. We will return to this later.

63

Fusing with the rules of experiential avoidance

In previous chapters we saw how experiential avoidance might be keeping you away from your values. We think that the processes of cognitive fusion that we have looked at in this chapter are a major cause of this experiential avoidance.

Suppose you evaluate your IBS experiences (bodily sensations, thoughts, memories or emotions) as something bad 'that will bring you harm'. When these experiences come up it is likely that you will do anything in your power to avoid them. You will create rules around your life to keep you from having these experiences because 'they will bring you harm'. You will make rules about not going out because you might have a symptom and feel embarrassed (and 'this will bring you harm'). You will make rules about not seeing people because they remind you of a healthier you that no longer exists (and 'that will bring you harm'). All sort of rules will be generated with the underlying imperative that the memories, the bodily sensations, the emotions and the thoughts related to IBS cannot be experienced because 'they will bring you harm'. This is the end result of cognitive fusion, when you identify with this overarching rule that experiences must be avoided because 'they will bring you harm'.

> **Right now as you read this book, try to notice if you are making rules about your life based on keeping thoughts and emotions related to IBS at bay. These rules often have a form of 'I should not ...', 'I would do ... but ...' or 'I won't be able to ... because ...' We will return to this later.**

Dealing with fusion or fused with the dealing?

By now your mind must be buzzing with all sorts of … you know it: thoughts! Probably you are thinking about how to deal with all this fusion mess or how to get rid of it. Your mind might be trying to come up with ways to change, eliminate or not think about these rules. Or it might be trying to find ways to not evaluate your IBS experiences or to evaluate them differently to your current process. Basically your mind is probably trying to find ways to control your thoughts or your feelings. This is the last level of fusion we need to address before we start working on how to distance yourself from your thoughts.

We get fused with the experiential avoidance way of solving problems. It is as if your car is broken: you approach this problem by trying to control it. You look at what is wrong with the car, and then you can take it to a mechanic, try to fix it yourself or even just get rid of it and buy a new one. This happens because we humans approach most things with a problem–solution model. If there is a problem, we fix it, change it or eliminate it. Because this approach works for about 90 per cent of our problems, we tend to become fused with this way of responding, much like the 'hammering away' example we talked about in the beginning of the chapter.

Now, this works fine if you are fixing your car, but it doesn't work as well when you are dealing with your feelings or your thoughts. Let's see if you can control your thoughts.

For the next few minutes try not to think of lemonade. Try not to think about its sweet taste or how refreshing it is on a hot summer day. Try not to think of its cloudy texture or how it feels going down your throat. Don't think about how your fingertips get numb from holding a cold glass of lemonade, or of all the moments in which you shared one with a friend or relative. You can think of anything else, just don't think of lemonade. Are you ready? Start.

Were you able not to think of lemonade?

Even if you didn't think of lemonade, how do you know you were not thinking of lemonade? You actually have to bring lemonade to your mind to know that you aren't thinking of it. If you try not thinking about something, or to think of it in a different way, you are actually bringing that thing to mind, whether it is lemonade, an unpleasant thought or a rule.

What about feelings? Society always tells us that we need to control the way we feel, as if that were a reasonable demand. Let's see how well that works.

Imagine for a moment that you are connected to the best anxiety detector in the world and that this detector is able to detect the slightest evidence of anxiety that you feel. If you have any feeling of anxiety a big red light will flash and we will know you are anxious. Now for this task we will ask you not to be anxious. And because we want you to succeed at this we have come up with a neat way to motivate you: we have another device connected to you that will give you a 10,000-volt shock if the red light flashes.

Now, what do you think will happen?

ZZZZZZZZZZZTTTTTTTTTTTT!!!!!!!!!!

That's right: you would probably be fried as soon as the anxiety detector was switched on.

These two exercises demonstrate the point that when it comes to your internal experiences, maybe experiential avoidance is probably not the best way to deal with them. When you approach your thoughts and feelings in a fused manner with this control/change/eliminate agenda you reduce the room for them to exist. But because they do exist and they don't go away, they just seem bigger, and because they are in a reduced space there seem to be more of them. We have a saying, which we will come back to and explain in a later chapter: 'If you are not willing to have it, you've got it.' Think about this and how it fits with what we have just discussed.

'So what can I do?' you might ask.

Defusion

So far we've seen how cognitive fusion can in certain situations promote actions that are not in line with your values, such as experiential avoidance. At this point we would like to present the alternative to cognitive fusion: cognitive defusion.

You will not find defusion in a dictionary; it is a new word coined by Acceptance and Commitment Therapy (ACT) therapists to describe the psychological event of looking *at* your thoughts rather than looking *from* your thoughts. When defused, you are able to watch your thoughts come and go without becoming attached to them. Defusion allows you to see thoughts for what they are: productions of your ever-buzzing mind. By defusing you are able to reclaim the driving wheel of your life rather than allowing your thoughts to dictate how you live. Defusion is not a trick, nor is it a form of eliminating or changing thoughts or emotions. It is not something that will remove your IBS, its symptoms, thoughts or feelings. It is not a form of getting away or hiding the pain deeper in your mind.

Defusion is a set of skills that you can learn that will give you enough distance from your thoughts so that you can make your choices without the influence of your mind. Remember from the previous chapter that your values orient the choices you make, and that sometimes choosing your values is difficult because your mind gets in the way. Learning to distance yourself from your thoughts can help you gain the perspective you need to choose the path of a valued life rather than the path of avoidance.

Coming back to the hammer example that we started this chapter with, defusion is a skill that will allow you to see that although you have a hammer in your hand, you also have several other tools, so the hammer is not the only solution even though your mind tells you so.

The following exercises are intended to undermine cognitive fusion and promote defusion. We encourage you to practise cognitive defusion as much as you can, because like any skill it is more effective if practised often. This does not mean that you should practise it all the time or that you should defuse completely from all the thoughts you have. After all, fusion is helpful sometimes — for example, you would not gain anything in defusing while trying to fix your car. We would like you to focus on the moments in which your mind drives you away from the choices that would lead you down the path of a life in line with your values.

Fusion diary

In order to gain a better view of the issues you are going to tackle in the defusion exercises that follow, it is essential that you take some time to find out exactly what you are struggling with. During this chapter, after each of the points we made on cognitive fusion we asked you to try to notice if you were engaging with these forms of fusion. We would now like you to take this a step further in an exercise designed to zero in on the aspects of fusion you are struggling with.

Exercise: Fusion diary

For the next week we would like you to focus on the thoughts you have that are related to your IBS. We would like you to notice and record the moments you engage in one or more forms of fusion, and what it leads to. So every time you notice a particular memory, prediction, evaluation, self-definition or rule coming up, note it in the appropriate space. Make a note, as well, of the situation you are in and what action your thoughts lead to. The intention of this exercise is not for you to try to change your thoughts or the outcomes in any way; for now we just want you to come into contact with the occurrence of these moments where fusion takes over. As you can see, the worksheet is divided into hourly segments. This doesn't mean you have to fill in every hour. For example, you won't be able to fill it in during the night while you are asleep. But if you wake up troubled by thoughts related to IBS you can jot them down there and then. We encourage you to carry this worksheet at all times; in the appendix of this book you will find several blank worksheets for you to photocopy. If you are in a situation in which it is not convenient to make a note, write it down as soon as you can. If you find that the worksheet is too small and you would like to make more notes than the space allows, feel free to use a diary or journal. If you feel a bit stuck starting, look at one of Angela's diary sheets (see pages 71–72).

Once you have completed a week of your fusion diary, come back to the book and continue working through this chapter.

FUSION DIARY			
Time	Situation	Thoughts (memory, prediction, evaluation, self-definition or rule)	Actions the thoughts lead to
1 am			
2 am			
3 am			
4 am			
5 am			
6 am			
7 am			
8 am			
9 am			
10 am			
11 am			
12 am			

table continued over page

Time	Situation	Thoughts (memory, prediction, evaluation, self-definition or rule)	Actions the thoughts lead to
1 pm			
2 pm			
3 pm			
4 pm			
5 pm			
6 pm			
7 pm			
8 pm			
9 pm			
10 pm			
11 pm			
12 pm			

When to use your mind, when to lose your mind

ANGELA'S FUSION DIARY			
Time	Situation	Thoughts (memory, prediction, evaluation, self-definition or rule)	Actions the thoughts lead to
1 am			
2 am			
3 am			
4 am			
5 am			
6 am			
7 am			
8 am	Woke up tired	The IBS is draining me.	Stayed in bed for an extra hour.
9 am	Having breakfast	I wish I could drink milk like I used to.	Couldn't eat any more.
10 am	Sitting on the sofa	I would be having my first class about now.	Cried
11 am	Still sitting around	I'm never going to get better.	Turned on the TV to drown this thought.
12 am	Lunch by myself	I am the loneliest person in the world.	Gobbled the rest of my lunch in a hurry.

table continued over page

Time	Situation	Thoughts (memory, prediction, evaluation, self-definition or rule)	Actions the thoughts lead to
1 pm	Phone call from my friend inviting me for coffee	I would like to go but I'm afraid there won't be an available toilet.	Refused the invitation.
2 pm	Going out to the shop for some cigarettes	Felt I wouldn't be able to make it.	Had to go to the loo three times to empty my bowels before leaving.
3 pm	Smoking a cigarette	I could be with my friend. Felt miserable for not being able to say yes.	Immediately lit up another to make myself feel better.
4 pm			
5 pm	My mum visited	I miss talking openly with my mum, but I'm too embarrassed.	Rushed out of the house and didn't pay much attention to what she told me.
6 pm			
7 pm	Preparing dinner	I cook all these healthy foods and I never feel better. Felt angry.	Threw the vegetables I was chopping across the room, making a mess.
8 pm	Watching TV	This is all I do all day.	Kept turning the TV on and off trying to decide what to do next.
9 pm	Turned off the TV	Felt really down and anxious. Need to get myself better to change my life.	Went to bed early.
10 pm			
11 pm			
12 pm			

Many people find this exercise hard to complete. Did you? It is hard to keep track of everything that is happening in our minds, and some thoughts about IBS tend to be muddled up with thoughts about other areas of our life. The main aim of this exercise was to come into contact with your thoughts about IBS. It is quite easy to have our lives dominated by thoughts when we are fused with our minds, and for us not to even notice that we are 'buying' all of these evaluations and judgements. With this diary you have now uncovered several situations in which you will be able to apply the following defusion skills.

Defusion skills

The following exercises will help you build a repertoire of skills that will allow you to gain some distance from your thoughts. Each exercise is very effective and can be used at any time. Although each targets a different area of fusion, they can be combined and used in situations where several layers of fusion are present.

Like training a muscle, defusion requires practice. To get the best results from the skills presented here, it is necessary that you practise them not only as you read this book but also in your everyday life. With continuing practice you might find that you can use your own ways to defuse from your thoughts, and even create your own exercises. In fact, many of the exercises ACT therapists use were created or inspired by the work done by their patients. So, anything you use that allows you to create some distance from your thoughts without trying to control them in any way could be considered a defusion technique.

Are you ready? Let's begin.

Exercise: Words, words, words

Language is a production of the mind and therefore likely to generate fusion. While jotting down your thoughts you might have noticed that certain words seem to have an enormous power over us. One word alone can start a chain reaction of painful thoughts. This happens because words have meaning for us; to speak or write them evokes an image or concept. When words pop into our heads it is hard to see them for what they are: just sounds or a collection of letters. Separating yourself from the meaning of painful words can alter your perspective.

A good way to gain some distance from this is to look at words the way you would if you were in a foreign country. In a place where you don't know the language it is hard to become attached to any meaning behind the sounds that the local people are making or the squiggly lines you see on a poster or newspaper.

For that to happen we are going to have to change the context of words, which can be done in many forms. Here are some suggestions.

Find a place where you can be alone, with no distractions. Take a few minutes and select a particular word or short form of thought with which you are struggling. It could be something like 'accident', 'IBS' or 'out of control'. Jot it down in the space below.

_____

Now write down any other thoughts and feelings that come attached to this word or short sentence.

_____
_____
_____

Now repeat that word aloud as quickly as you can for a minute. Just keep saying your chosen word over and over again. Start now!

How was that for you? Did you notice anything different happening to the word you chose? Did it still have the same effect on you? Did it bring up the same negative psychological content?

Maybe it started to sound different or strange. Maybe your mouth felt funny from the movements. Maybe it sounded a bit like a song or a chant. Many people find that the negative content in the word they choose seems to become detached from the word itself.

Try the same exercise with other words or thoughts that cause you pain. You can also try all sorts of vocalisations; you don't have to stick to 'quickly' as we suggested. You can try saying it very slowly or, as unusual as it sounds, you can sing the word. You can also say it in a different voice, altering the pitch from low to high. Try to imitate the word as if it were being said by someone else — Donald Duck or George W. Bush. Even if you think this is a silly idea, we urge you to try it out just a few times and simply notice what effect it has on your experience of the words.

Exercise: Labelling your experiences

One way to gain some distance and see your thoughts for what they are — just thoughts — is to call them by their names. Instead of thinking the thoughts, why don't you call out what you are doing? Thinking, 'I'm feeling anxious' is quite different from, 'I am having the feeling of anxiety.' See if you can apply labelling to your experiences. Applying a label would look something like this:

* I am having the thought that … (describe your thought)
* I am having the feeling of … (describe your feeling)
* I am having the memory of … (describe your memory)
* I am making the prediction of … (describe your prediction)
* I am having the bodily sensation of … (describe the bodily sensation)
* I am making the rule of … (describe your rule)

For a couple of minutes just let your experiences flow. While doing this jot down below how you would label your experiences. If you are willing, try saying these statements aloud. That can help you to see them as they are. Remember that even, 'I'm not having any experience' can be 'I am having the thought that I am not having any experience.'

_____

_____

_____

_____

_____

_____

_____

_____

_____

This was just a practice run. The challenge now is for you to try to use this in your everyday life. See if you can devote some moments of your day to labelling your experiences. Start with situations in which you are not distressed, and gradually introduce labelling into distressing situations.

Exercise: Buses on the street

This will be an eyes-closed exercise. Read the instructions, and when you feel you are ready, start the exercise.

Imagine that you are standing on the footpath of a busy street. There is a lot of noise and people going everywhere. In front of you an endless parade of double-decker buses goes by. Each of these buses has a space for advertising.

Once you have this image in your head, try to become conscious of your thoughts. Each time a thought comes up mentally place it in the advertising space of the bus. If you think in words, imagine each thought as a slogan on the side of the bus; if you think in pictures, imagine them as a poster for an upcoming movie. Try to keep yourself on the footpath looking at your thoughts going by on the buses. Don't try to make the buses go faster or slower, or to change what is on the advertising space. If the buses disappear, if you find yourself on the bus or if you walk away from the footpath to go somewhere else, just stop and notice this, then file that knowledge and return to the footpath to look at some more thoughts.

Do this for at least five minutes. It is useful to keep a watch close by. Are you ready to give it a shot? Begin!

How long did it take until the buses stopped or disappeared, or you went somewhere else or boarded the bus? What happened just before you got caught up by your thoughts?

You can think of the moments you got caught up in your thoughts as moments of cognitive fusion. At those points you stopped looking *at* your thoughts and started looking *from* your thoughts. The moments in which you were able to stay on the footpath looking at the buses can be considered moments of cognitive defusion. This exercise often leads to thoughts like, 'I'm not doing this right' or 'This doesn't work for me.' It is quite easy to become fused with these thoughts and stop the exercise. Why not take notice of these thoughts and stick them on the side of the bus?

Repeating this exercise regularly will enable you to stay on the footpath for longer just looking at your thoughts going by on the buses. Repeating the exercise helps to make the defusion process easier. It is not a goal to achieve five minutes of defusion — even Zen masters have great difficulty in staying with this exercise and need to bring themselves back to the footpath several times.

Exercise: Where do I sit?

If you are reading this book, odds are that you are sitting somewhere in a chair or on a sofa or a stool. We would like you to take a couple of minutes to think of where you are sitting, and then jot down as many characteristics as you can come up with for it.

_____

_____

_____

_____

_____

Let's take the example of a sofa. While sitting in a sofa we could come up with things such as: 'It's brown', 'It has two large cushions', 'It weighs a lot' and 'It has four wooden feet'. All these characteristics are part of the primary attributes that we can see in the sofa. They are a description of what can be directly observed in the sofa. What we mean is that no matter who looks at this sofa, these characteristics will not change.

But we could have just as easily said, 'This is a good sofa', 'It is comfortable', 'We like the colour of it'. These would be evaluations that we would be making about the sofa, and therefore secondary characteristics of the sofa. These would depend on our interaction with the sofa and all our previous history with sofas. For example, we evaluate it as being comfortable because we can compare it to previous sofas we have sat on, but 'comfortable' will not be a primary characteristic of the sofa, since someone else could find it uncomfortable.

Odds are that in your attempt to offer a _description_ of where you are sitting you have probably added some _evaluations_ as well.

Remember that evaluations are a particularly sticky subject when it comes to fusion. When you are evaluating where you sit, it has no great bearing on your actions; the most that can happen is for you to try to find another place to sit if this is too uncomfortable. But when it comes to our experiences (events, bodily sensations, feelings and thoughts), evaluations can be quite troublesome. Much of our suffering comes from this confusion between descriptions and evaluations. Quite often we see our evaluations as being primary properties of the experiences we are having and act according to them.

Doing this is quite hard and it is probably more obvious for an object (such as where you are sitting) than it is for our private experiences. So let's try to get there gradually in the form of this exercise.

Try to list some attributes for a table in your home:

Descriptions: (colour, material, etc.)

_____

_____

Evaluations: (good, bad, practical, pretty, etc.)

_____

_____

Now try to do the same for a friend of yours:

Descriptions: (height, hair colour, eye colour, etc.)

_____

_____

_____

Evaluations: (close friend, beautiful, ugly, good, etc.)

_____

_____

_____

Now try to do the same for an IBS experience. Think about the last bout you had and list the properties of that experience in the same way you did for a table or your friend. For example, someone who had a severe bout of diarrhoea with great anxiety might list 'loose stools', 'light-headedness' or 'heart pounding' as descriptions, while 'This was the worst experience of my life' or 'The embarrassment was unbearable' could be listed as evaluations of the event.

Descriptions:

_____

_____

_____

Evaluations:

_____

_____

Now try to bring this to your everyday life as well. Try to catch yourself in the evaluations you make. In difficult situations try to see if you are relating to the experience itself or the evaluation of the experience. Being able to distinguish between descriptions and evaluations should allow you to have some more space to move in the direction you want no matter how your mind evaluates the situation you are in.

Exercise: Kicking your buts

The use of the word 'but' in sentences has the function of creating an opposition between two statements. When you say, 'I would like to go out to eat *but* my IBS might flare up', the word 'but' functions as a statement that 'going out to eat' and 'my IBS might flare up' cannot happen at the same time.

Go back to your fusion diary and see if you have some 'but' statements there, or take a couple of days to jot down some 'but' statements in the spaces below. If it is difficult for you to find these statements, think of your values and see if there are any 'buts' keeping you from going in the direction you really want to take.

_____ but _____

_____ but _____

_____ but _____

_____ but _____

_____ but _____

_____ but _____

_____ but _____

_____ but _____

_____ but _____

_____ but _____

Now see what happens when you take the same sentences and change the word 'but' to the word 'and'.

_____ and _____

_____ and _____

_____ and _____

_____ and _____

_____ and _____

_____ and _____

_____ and _____

_____ and _____

_____ and _____

Did you notice any difference? Are the 'and' sentences less believable than the 'but' sentences? How was the meaning of the sentence affected and how can that be important to you?

Let's look at our example: 'I would like to go out to eat _but_ my IBS might flare up.' By changing it to an 'and' sentence, it will become: 'I would like to go out to eat _and_ my IBS might flare up.' By using the word 'and', suddenly going out to eat and having an IBS flare-up can actually coexist. Aren't both of these statements true? The difference is that the second one allows you to contemplate the choice of going out to eat while the first one automatically excludes this. Now think of all the times that IBS-related thoughts, bodily sensations or feelings following a 'but' excluded you from the possibility of contemplating whatever came before that 'but'. Think of how that affected your life.

Take this idea into the real world and try to catch yourself making these 'but' statements. See if replacing 'but' with 'and' works as well as — and sometimes even better — in certain situations.

'If I'm not my thoughts who am I?'

The quote in this heading is from an ACT client who posed this question to his therapist.[1] And you might have had this feeling while working through this chapter: that we are not what we produce in our minds. We are much more. This is the issue we will address in the next chapter. We will also show you how to take these defusion skills to a different level by learning how to stay in contact with the present moment with a skill called mindfulness.

CHAPTER 6

Mindfulness — a new perspective

In the previous chapter we addressed the problems of fusion and how to gain a different perspective on some of the things that your 'mind' says, in order to undermine the role of the mind when we have to make choices that are related to our values. The defusion techniques we taught you do not focus on ways of changing your IBS experiences but rather on ways of being able to observe them. Observing your experiences can be an empowering and scary place to be. On one hand it can help you gain some perspective so that you see more choices in key situations and on the other hand it can put you in touch with these painful experiences that you have been working so hard to avoid. Also, as we noticed at the end of the previous chapter, being in this position raises the question: If your mind is one of the things being observed, who is doing the observing?

There are two key elements to be addressed in this chapter. The first is to define and put you in touch with this observing self. This will give you a perspective of yourself from which you can be in contact with your painful IBS experiences and still choose to move in your valued directions. The second element to be addressed is how to use mindfulness to harness this perspective in the present moment. Possessing this skill can help you look at your experiences in a less entangled way while remaining in contact with the present moment. This will allow you to choose to move in your valued direction even if in the short term it will put you in touch with painful experiences.

So let's start by looking at what we mean by 'the observing self'.

Me, myself and I

Throughout this book we have spent a lot of time talking about your 'self'. But what do we mean by this?

Although there are many definitions of 'self' and several ways of understanding your experiences, we will stick to three: the conceptualised self, the self as ongoing awareness and the observer self.

Having a better understanding of these senses of self is crucial to achieving a perspective from which you are able to develop a firm sense of who you are and what you want to stand for (your values), while at the same time being defused from your thoughts. By understanding these senses of self you can move from the identification you are making with your conceptualised self to identifying with your observing self.

Let's have a closer look at what we mean by these different selves.

The conceptualised self

The conceptualised self is the way we see ourselves through our mind's eye. It is the distilled product that our mind gives us from all our history, evaluations, memories, thoughts, feelings and bodily sensations that tells us who and what we are. To put it simply, it is the picture we carry of ourselves.

The way we see ourselves can take many shapes and forms depending on the way we judge our own personal story. Some of us think of ourselves in a positive light: 'I am a friendly person' or 'I am an organised person.' Some of us carry a more negative picture: 'I am a failure as a person' or 'I am an anxious person.' You probably saw some of these coming up in the 'I am ...' exercise in the previous chapter. Whether the label is negative or positive, the fact is that it can greatly impact the way we live our life.

One of the self-conceptualisations that is frequent with IBS patients is, 'I am a person with IBS.' Perhaps you wrote something like this in the 'I am ...' exercise. When you describe yourself in this way your conceptualised self is at work, choosing one particular part of your history to define you. This doesn't mean that this statement is untrue; after all, if you are reading this book you are indeed someone who has IBS. The thing is that when this becomes a key issue in the way you tell your life story, everything else seems to get tainted by it.

For example, imagine you are faced with the prospect of going out to lunch with your friend. It would be common for your mind to tell you, 'I am a person who has IBS; I'm not sure I'll be able to go; what if I have an accident?' This element of your story is likely to dominate over other aspects of your story such as, 'I am a person capable of walking to the restaurant,' 'I am a friend,' 'I am a person who enjoys food.' Frequently, you end up not going because you are 'a person who has IBS'.

We are not suggesting that the conceptualised self is in some sense untrue or unhelpful. For example, if you are an accountant and you are not able to identify yourself with this self-conceptualisation while doing your job, you might find it hard to experience a sense of confidence in your working role. But identifying with 'I am an accountant' while playing football on a sunny Sunday afternoon might not be very useful to score goals.

We are not asking you to get rid of the ways you conceptualise yourself. Instead, we would like you to notice that you are much more than what your mind tells you. You have IBS, yes, and you are also many other things. Conceptualisations are part of who you are but they are not 'you'.

Self as ongoing awareness

Ongoing self-awareness is a continuous and fluid contact with the experiences you have in the present moment. It is those moments in which you are aware of what is happening exactly as it is and not as it says it is. It is like the conceptualised self because you still use verbal categories to describe it, and it is also different in the sense that it does not judge or evaluate, it just describes. For example, it is when you notice, 'I am thinking this,' 'I am feeling that,' 'I am tasting this' or 'I am remembering that.' This is the self that gives you a sense of personal history, a sense of who you are in time. It is like a record of your experiences without the entanglement of evaluations.

Because of these qualities of conceptualisation and defusion that occur at the same time, this sense of self can be a double-edged sword.

Being aware of what happened to you at a certain point in time can be helpful in socialisation. You can remember an event you experienced with a friend and share the memory of that event over a chat, going through the description of the event. In the same way it is also helpful to know your history with IBS. Objective facts about your experience with IBS can be shared with your family, friends and doctor. The memory of the first IBS bout you ever had can hold valuable information about which symptoms you have, when they started and how they appeared. As long as you keep this descriptive sense without going into evaluations and judgements about the facts, this sense of self is very consistent with a defused way of being.

We humans, however, have a tendency to judge our history and use labels to describe events. For example, you could view the first time you had a bout of IBS as the worst day of your life. Although it is understandable that you see it that way, it is just that — the way *you* view it. It does not make the description of the event any more accurate. When you buy into the evaluations your mind produces for these events, you are adding a judgement to your story and the way you tell it. Therefore you are contributing to your conceptualised self.

The observing self

One way to define the observing self is to say that it is the 'you' that is looking behind your eyes. It is the 'you' that has been present since you were born until today and that has observed every change in between.

These are very rough definitions because it is hard to put into words something that is not quantifiable and that does not have a shape. The observing self is something that can only be experienced. To make a bit more sense of this, it is useful to use an exercise that will get you in touch with this sense of self. During this exercise you may only catch a glimpse of what we are describing. That is enough, the self as observer is not something we can hold, but we can get moments of contact with it.

Exercise: Looking for the observing self

In this exercise we would like you to read each point at a time and then to close your eyes and try to immerse yourself as deeply as you can in the action requested. After that, come back to the book and jot down what came up for you and then continue to the next point.

1. Try to notice what is happening right now. Close your eyes and take note of any sounds or smells that come to you. Notice how the material you are sitting on feels against your body. Notice any thoughts, feelings, bodily sensations or memories. Do this for about thirty seconds and then come back to the book.

While jotting down what you became aware of in the space below, try to understand who was doing the noticing.

_____

_____

_____

_____

_____

_____

_____

2. Now try to think of something that happened in the past six months. It doesn't have to be a good or a bad event; it just has to be something that sticks out in your mind. Once you have chosen an event try to get back to that moment and see if you can mentally slip into your skin again. Close your eyes and see if you can notice what was happening then, what you saw, the sounds, the smells, the tastes, what you thought about it, what you felt. Do this for about thirty seconds and then come back to the book.

While jotting down what you became aware of in the space below, again try to understand who was doing the noticing.

_____

_____

_____

_____

_____

_____

_____

_____

3. Now try to remember an event from your teen years. Again, it doesn't matter if it is good or bad. Just close your eyes and try to step into that memory as if you were there again and try to notice what was going on: the sights, smells, bodily sensations, sounds, thoughts and feelings. Do this for thirty seconds and then come back to the book.

While jotting down what you became aware of in the space below, again try to understand who was doing the noticing.

_____

_____

_____

_____

_____

_____

_____

Now try to answer this question: Where were 'you' in all these situations?

You might have noticed that now, six months ago and several years ago there was only one person noticing what was happening: 'you'. That is your observing self. In a very real and important way you have been you for the whole of your life. Somehow this 'you' connects all these situations and remains unchanged in some way. If you notice, this self is the same person that observed your experiences as a teen although your body, your roles, your thoughts and your feelings have changed. This self encompasses all your history and experiences and yet it is not bound to them. It is not bound to the conceptualisations that you made then or that you make now, it just watches you make them. This self is timeless because it has been there since you were born. You can't get away from it, because wherever you go, there 'you' are. Because it cannot be separated from you it is probably the most complete representation of who you are.

Some people find it very hard to come into contact with this self because they are still very attached (fused) to the way their mind perceives the world. Their mind immediately tries to come up with solutions to resolve this conundrum.

Maybe the sum of my memories defines who I am

Memories work a lot like snippets of film. Even if you were able to collate all these snippets into a huge masterpiece, would that be you? Probably not, because the observing 'you' was the one who captured those snippets. In a way the observing 'you' is the director who was behind the camera filming.

Maybe my thoughts and feelings define who I am

Although our thoughts and feelings are a great part of our experience, who is doing the thinking and feeling and noticing it? Thoughts and feelings change constantly. Thus you are more than just your thoughts and feelings. Throughout your life you change the way you feel and think about things all the time. And still there is someone observing these changes.

Maybe my roles define who I am

Have you ever thought of how many roles you adopt throughout your life? For example, son/daughter, father/mother, student/employee, shopper/seller. Even throughout the day you can be the breakfast maker, the driver, the employee, the friend, the husband/wife, go back to being the driver ... thus you are more than just your roles. Situations change, and your roles change with them, and still there is always someone there to pick up every new role, and that someone doesn't change: the observing self.

Maybe my body defines who I am

There's nothing like some solid evidence of our existence to make sense of things! Our bodies exist, therefore that is how we can limit and define our observer self — after all, if the body ceases to exist the observer self ceases to exist. Or does it? If you think about it, your body is completely different now to what it was when you were born. Your body was different as a toddler, a child, a teenager and as an adult. You might have gained scars, wrinkles or moles that were not there fifteen years ago. Your entire skin changes every six weeks. All the cells in your body are replaced by new cells within the space of seven years. Each year 95 per cent of the atoms in your body are replaced. And still, there 'you' are, observing.

What is the purpose of all this?

Gaining contact with your observing self is a powerful place to be. You know that 'you' will continue, no matter what happens, even though your mind tells you 'this will bring you harm' (remember the previous chapter?). Being the observer puts you in a position from which whatever is going on at that moment is not good, bad, scary or dangerous, it is just another experience that you can register. This creates a space in which it is okay to have difficult and painful IBS experiences. We don't mean you have to like them (that is an evaluation), what we mean is that you *can* have them. Now think of the impact this can have on your choices. If you look from your observing-self perspective, could it be possible to *have* your IBS experiences and still move in a vital and valued direction? Could it be possible to have a life that is about your values and still have your IBS experiences? Being able to carry these difficult IBS experiences releases you from the conditions of having to get rid of IBS before you move forward on the path you value. The next exercise will help make this clearer.

Exercise: The planet of you

Imagine that your life is a planet floating around in a galaxy, and that this planet is inhabited by immortal creatures. Each of these creatures represents your life experiences such as your thoughts, feelings, bodily sensations and memories. Although these creatures are all different they tend to hang around with those that are more similar to them, and they tend to divide into tribes.

Let's say that regarding your IBS you have two tribes: the positive tribe and the negative tribe. Like most radically different tribes, these two have been at war for a long time. On one side is the negative tribe with all your uncomfortable bodily sensations from the IBS symptoms; all your painful IBS-related memories; all your worries, anxiety, sadness about your IBS; all your fears about an uncertain life with IBS; and many more. On the other side you have the positive tribe with the happiness of a day without symptoms; the wish to gain back control of your life; feelings of confidence; and many other positive experiences you have related to your IBS.

Like in all wars the objective of each side is to win. So in these endless battles the two tribes go at each other trying to eliminate the adversary. But remember that these creatures are immortal so they never really eliminate one another. Sometimes they can push one of their enemies out to the side of the battlefield, but they are still on the same planet and eventually they find their way back to the battlefront. And because they are your experiences they just keep increasing their numbers every day you live, on each side. These tribes will keep battling away for an eternity, so relentless are they in their efforts to eliminate one another.

Some days you'll have a good day and it will seem that the positive tribe gained some territory and was able to get the negative tribe out of the field of battle. Other days it will seem like the negative tribe took control of the whole planet and all the negative experiences of your IBS seem to be in your face.

Being the General

Most of us spend our lives being the General for the positive tribe. We devise several strategies to win this war. Sometimes we decide on a full-frontal attack to have our positive experiences overcome our negative experiences. Sometimes, because the other side has grown in size or their members look scarier and bigger than usual, our strategy is to retreat and avoid the battle. But as we have seen, no matter what strategy you use, the war will continue. Whether you support one side or the other, the direction of your life remains dependent on the outcome of the battle.

Now we ask you, if you keep battling every day, are you really moving anywhere? Does supporting either side make it possible to move on with your life? And where are you in all of this? Are you one of the Generals? Maybe you are one of the members of the tribe? Try to think of this and write your thoughts in the space below.

_____

_____

_____

_____

_____

In this exercise many people realise that they spend most of their time choosing a side or devising a strategy — but don't you contain both sides of this battle? Aren't you both the positive and negative Generals? And what does that mean? Every member of both these tribes is a part of you. When they fight, what is really happening? Aren't you fighting yourself? Going to war with yourself can only have one outcome: you will always be in a fight!

IBS is a part of who you are, and every time you try to fight it you are actually fighting yourself. Every battle you engage in is a losing one, no matter who wins. And the biggest problem is that this war doesn't end. When you see IBS as your enemy that has to be eliminated you simply perpetuate this war. Now, do you really want to live in constant battle?

But what if you are neither side in this war? What if you are not for or against your IBS? What if you can contain these experiences? Who are you then?

Being the planet

As we see it, you are the planet on which this war has been raging for years. You are not on the positive or the negative side; you contain both sides. Being the planet is what we mean by being the observing self. The planet contains both positive and negative tribes and their Generals, just like you contain both positive and negative experiences related to your IBS.

If you look from the planet perspective you need not choose sides, because no matter what happens in the battles you will always contain every tribe member. Looking from this perspective, in which you can hold both sides without engaging in the battle, is what we call being in the 'observing self' seat.

The importance of being a planet

As we have seen, one of the most important things a planet can do is to hold all the positive and negative tribes (IBS experiences) without becoming entangled in the ongoing war between them. Another thing a planet can do is to move while carrying the tribes. Now, think about the importance of these two characteristics. What would it mean in terms of your life with IBS if you could carry your experiences, positive and negative, and still move in any direction? And in what direction would you move?

By now you are probably seeing more clearly where we are going with this. Being in the observer seat enables you to move in any direction while carrying your experiences, which means that going in the direction of your values is *not* dependent on how you feel (physically and psychologically) or think. It means that you can take your difficult experiences with you while you pursue directions that make your life more meaningful. From this perspective, if a scary experience comes up it need not affect your movement in a valued direction, it is just something else you are taking with you for the ride. This is not a trick; when a scary thing comes up, it will still be scary. You will likely still experience the same sensations and fears and thoughts you have always experienced. What we ask is that you notice the experiences that your mind and body are giving you, and see them as experiences rather than reasons to do something. We also ask that you notice all of these from the perspective of the 'you' that has lived through your whole life, and that you continue to take steps, however small or large, towards what you most value, and that you bring the scary experiences along with you.

Mindfulness

Being mindful is the ability to be in contact with all your personal experiences (good or bad) in the present moment, observing them and not buying the judgements that your mind will make of them. You can see this is more or less what we aimed to do in the 'Buses on the street' exercise in Chapter 5. In fact, mindfulness is like an older cousin of defusion, and like defusion it needs to be practised. In the rest of this chapter we will focus on how to make mindfulness a part of your life, so that in those difficult moments when you struggle with your IBS experiences you can approach them from the perspective of the observing self. This will help you make those vital and valued choices without being entangled in the content of the war playing out in your life.

Mindfulness practice

As you begin to experience more and more of this observing sense of self, it will probably be easier for you to just sit with your experiences no matter how they look or feel. Being mindful implies accessing this sense of self in the here and now. So, being mindful is actually quite simple, it is just a question of paying attention to what is happening at this moment.

There are many things we can be mindful of, and we have included a few exercises and techniques that are particularly relevant to IBS. But before we begin we would like to say a few words about the practice of mindfulness.

When?

The ultimate goal is to practise mindfulness at any time wherever you are. But like any good skill this needs to be developed at your own pace. Because you are just starting it is preferable that you schedule a particular part of the day to the practice of mindfulness.

Also, it is better if you start with just two or three times per week and then build up from there. You can set aside, say, ten minutes on each of these days to practise mindfulness, and build up from there as well. If this seems a bit much for you, think of how much time you spend struggling with your IBS. If you add all the time you dedicate to thinking, battling, trying to eliminate or control IBS, isn't that much more than three half-hour sessions in a week?

When you are more comfortable with this practice, try to extend it to the remaining days of the week. Mindfulness is not about practising only when you have planned to do it. If you find moments in your day where the opportunity presents itself to practise mindfulness (and there are always opportunities), just go for it.

Because mindfulness involves meditation exercises, many people think of it as a relaxation technique. But mindfulness is not about finding relaxation — if you do, that is fine, but if you don't, that is fine too. The point is to be consciously aware of what is happening, not to try to change it.

Some people believe that if they feel bad, psychologically or physically, they should not practise mindfulness, but mindfulness can be practised no matter how you feel. In some of the mindfulness exercises, negative content is bound to appear, and this is just another experience to take notice of. Feeling too bad to practise mindfulness is just another evaluation that your mind is giving you, something that could be noticed in your practice.

Where?

Ideally you will be able to practise mindfulness wherever you are, but it is advisable that initially you find a place where you won't be distracted. Distractions are part of the mindfulness practice and are regarded as more experiences that you can notice, but it is probably easier to do this once you have developed your skills in a quieter environment. So when you are making your schedule it might be helpful to decide where you can practise for ten minutes without being interrupted.

How?

Just be in the here and now! It is as simple as that. Mindfulness is about sitting in the observing-self seat and watching your experiences. Sometimes it will feel easy, and sometimes it will feel hard to do it. Sometimes you might experience symptoms, sometimes you won't. You'll come into contact with positive and negative experiences. All these are part of the things you can notice in a defused way.

Mindfulness is not about experiencing some sort of mystical or peaceful state. You are not trying to get into a trance, you are simply coming into contact with what you observe in a moment-to-moment manner.

You will probably make judgements about whether you are doing this mindfulness thing right or wrong. Mindfulness is not another standard for you to judge yourself by. It is not about success or failure. If you end up having these doubts running through your mind, just notice them and keep noticing what comes up in each moment.

Let's begin the exercises!

Exercise: Right here, right now

Below is a set of instructions that will help you become mindfully aware of what is happening around and in you, in the present moment. You can either memorise the instructions or record them and have them played back to you while you practise this exercise. This script is just a suggestion and you can adapt it to better fit you as long as you keep the basic components of focusing your attention on what is happening now.

Wherever you are — sitting on a chair, or lying on the floor or a bed — find a comfortable position in which you can stay throughout the exercise.

Now take a moment to look around and notice what is surrounding you. Look at each object, notice it and then move to the next one. After doing this, focus on something that caught your eye. It might be a point on a wall, a particular object, a particular sight. Try to stay focused on that for the remainder of the exercise.

Now tune into the sounds you can hear. Are there any particular sounds that stand out? Maybe you can hear what is happening on the street, maybe what's happening in the next room or just the electric hum of the lights. Is there a particular sound that catches your attention? Do you notice yourself thinking whether this is a nice or unpleasant sound? Just try to notice that evaluation and go back to noticing the sounds in the room.

Now smell what is around you. How does it smell where you are right now? Can you actually sense any smell? If you do, does this smell remind you of anything? Note what comes up in your mind when you notice that particular smell. Are you still here? If you drift off to some memory or thought, bring yourself back to this moment.

Now pay attention to your body. Is there any particular area of your body that you are more aware of than others? How does that feel? Try to notice that and then move on to your fingertips. Rub them together. How does that feel? Can you feel your fingerprints? Do your hands feel rough or smooth? Now try to notice the places in your body that are in contact with whatever you are sitting or lying on. Can you notice anything about the surface your body is in contact with? Can you feel the shape of the points in which your body makes contact with these surfaces? How does that make you feel? Just notice it and then let it go.

Now bring your focus to your belly. Are you feeling any discomfort? We are just having a look, so don't be scared. Are you feeling any of your IBS symptoms? How does that feel? Try to make a note of it. Even if you are not feeling any discomfort, how does focusing on your belly feel to you? Does it bring up uncomfortable thoughts, feelings or memories? Try to notice them and then let them go. If you find yourself being pulled by a bodily sensation, a thought or feeling, bring yourself back gently and try to watch it go by in front of you. Don't forget it is part of who you are.

Now try to notice what you are feeling. Any particular feelings? Do you feel scared or anxious about your IBS? If so, just notice 'you are having the feeling of anxiety' and as best you can, allow it to be there without holding on to it or needing it to go away. Are you remembering embarrassing moments related to IBS? You can watch them too. Just be the planet and welcome every member of every tribe.

Now turn to your thoughts. What is your mind giving you today? A sentence that repeats over and over again? How does that sound? Maybe a picture that comes to your mind in vivid colours and detail? How does that look? Try to notice your mind doing its never-ending work of producing thoughts.

Is this exercise taking you anywhere in the past to a difficult memory? Maybe it is going in the opposite direction to a predicted future? If you find yourself thinking of the past or future you may notice that you have been pulled away from the immediate experience. If you do notice this, it is an opportunity to simply notice what it was that drew your attention away and then gently let it go and bring your attention back to the here and now.

This exercise has no specific end or duration. You can keep noticing whatever is around or within you. If you feel like you've finished, bring yourself back to where you are and notice that you were here and now for a moment. Go back to the rest of your day.

Exercise: Daily mindfulness exercises

We will now focus on several mindfulness exercises that can be incorporated in your daily activities. Remember, every moment is an opportunity to be mindful.

Mindful eating

This can be a very touchy subject for people with IBS since many people pay a lot of attention to what they eat. So it might come as a surprise that we would like you to incorporate mindfulness into your meals. With all the attention and care you put into the food you eat, have you set aside some time to really notice the process of eating?

Take your time to have your meal. Go through it slowly, paying attention to every action you make. Notice the movements of your hands while the cutlery slices the food. When you bite it, notice the smell, the flavour and the textures as it swirls around in your mouth.

While you eat, are there any thoughts, feelings or bodily sensations coming up? Try to simply notice them too.

Are you eating alone? Are you eating with someone you know or in the middle of strangers? Watch what comes up in these different situations, and how your mind reacts.

Just like any other moment, eating can be used as a way to come into contact with who you are in the here and now.

Mindfulness in your morning routine

Pick an activity in your daily routine, such as brushing your teeth, washing your face or having a shower, and try every day to focus on this activity. Notice what you are doing: the body movements, the smells, the sounds.

Let's take brushing your teeth as an example. Bring your focus to how the tap feels as you turn it on. Notice the sound of the water running. Notice if it is hot or cold. Feel the weight and touch of the toothbrush as you hold it. Catch the smell of the toothpaste as you open the tube. Focus on the feeling the brush produces against your teeth, against the sides of your mouth. Notice how your tongue moves around. Notice the taste of the toothpaste and the slight burning sensation of the mint. Focus on the feeling around your mouth as you swish the water and spit it out.

If thoughts or feelings arise during this, acknowledge them, let them be, and bring your attention back to your brushing. Your attention is likely to wander. When this happens, make a note of it and then bring yourself back to what you are doing.

Mindfulness in your domestic chores

Pick any domestic activity, such as ironing your clothes, vacuuming the floor or washing the dishes, and try to do it mindfully.

Let's take the example of washing the dishes. Notice the temperature of the water, the feeling of the washing-up liquid against your skin. Focus on the smells of both the dirty dishes and the washing-up liquid. Notice how the crumbly textures and the colours on the plates disappear as you scrub them. Notice the movements of your arms and hands during this process.

If any feelings or thoughts arise, just notice them and then bring yourself back to the task. Again, your attention might start to wander to memories or to plans about what you will be doing next. Just notice them and continue to focus on this activity.

Exercise: Sitting

This is one of the oldest and most popular forms of mindfulness practice. The key to it is: just sit. Nothing else. Sounds easy, doesn't it? But like many simple things it can be quite tricky to do.

This is not a meditation or spiritual exercise; it is just another opportunity to watch what unfolds in our minds.

Dedicate a moment of your day to this practice. You can start with just five or ten minutes and gradually build up to larger amounts of time.

Find a comfortable place to sit. When you sit it is very important to take care with your posture. If you are sitting on a chair make sure your back is straight and relaxed, and that you are not leaning against the back of the chair. Do not cross your legs; try to keep your knees shoulder-width apart. If you are sitting on the floor or on a cushion on the floor, there are many combinations of leg postures you can use. You can have them crossed in many ways or just slightly arched in front of you. Whatever makes it possible and comfortable for you to maintain good back posture as described above will be fine. Finally, rest your hands in your lap (one on top of the other, palms down) and keep your arms slightly away from your trunk.

The purpose of the exercise is to remain in the sitting position for the period of time you have set yourself, so once you have achieved a stable and steady posture try to move as little as possible for the duration of the exercise.

Begin by focusing on your breathing. Notice how it feels for the air to pass in and out of your lungs, through your throat, your nose; how warm it is when it comes out.

Then bring your attention to your body. While sitting still you will begin to feel discomfort. Don't be alarmed; this is part of human nature and physiology. You will have the urge to move, squirm or change position — unless you really have to move, try to stay in the sitting position. Try to just notice and embrace your discomfort as part of yourself.

We are not saying that you should not move at all. If you feel you can't endure it, give yourself a break; you can try again after this or leave it for next time. But remember to notice what is going on while you break from the posture — are you following a rule or a particular thought or sensation?

This is a great opportunity to see your mind at work trying to come up with solutions to eliminate your discomfort. Try to notice if anything comes to your mind, such as reasons to move or rationalisations to break away from the exercise. Notice these thoughts and then let them go while remaining in the same position.

Also, during the exercise you might notice difficult thoughts or feelings, some of which are related to your IBS. Some of them might even come up in the reasons your mind is giving you to stop the exercise, such as: 'My stomach is rumbling, I am afraid I might need to go to the bathroom.' Try to hold these thoughts and feelings and still remain seated until the end of the exercise.

Being able to go through this exercise can be a powerful experience because you will be in contact with your observing self throughout it. You will be able to watch and hold your experiences even if they are uncomfortable. But most importantly, by being able to sit with your discomfort you are creating a space in which discomfort is another part of your experience that does not have to dictate your choices. With practice this will set a precedent that you can then take into your daily life. Imagine being able to sit with your discomfort in real life and still move in the direction you most value. Now, that sounds like a moving planet capable of holding its tribes!

Mindfulness and willingness

Mindfulness is very powerful because it can change the perspective you have about your IBS, which in turn can open new doors and alternatives for how to relate to your symptoms, thoughts and feelings. In itself this is very helpful, but we want more. As we have said, this book is about living your life the way you most want it to be lived. It is time now to take these skills and make use of them to get you back to the directions you explored in your values work. The last exercise of this chapter already touched the core of what we will talk about in the next chapter: willingness. In fact, it was a good introduction to how you could make use of these mindfulness skills so that you can willingly come into contact with your IBS experiences while still moving in the directions you most value. We are talking about living *with* IBS rather than having a life dictated by IBS.

So, if you are willing to give this a chance, read on!

CHAPTER 7

Are you willing to have IBS?

In Chapter 3 we saw that trying to control your symptoms and the stress associated with them was, in many cases, leading you away from the life you would like to live. We suggested that this controlling/avoiding/eliminating agenda, although logical, was not the most workable way to deal with IBS suffering.

Remember when we compared the situation you are living in to a pit of quicksand, with all those gooey IBS symptoms, feelings and thoughts? We suggested that the most likely approach you had been taking so far had been to try to fight your way out of the quicksand. We also saw how such fighting is actually counterproductive, because the more you try to struggle to get out, the more entangled you become. But we offered a solution as well: to get out of actual quicksand you have to get as much of your body into contact with the sand as possible. With this in mind, we suggest that the way out of your IBS suffering could come from getting *more* in touch with your experiences, as unpleasant as they are, and having them while still moving in the direction you really want to go.

This chapter is about taking the first step to doing exactly that. We will ask that instead of trying to fight your way out of your IBS experiences, you voluntarily and willingly come into contact with them, fully embracing them as a part of your experience that can come along for this ride that we call life.

For this, the skills of defusion and mindfulness we have been working on so far will be essential. Also essential is having your values present so that they can point the way.

What is acceptance/willingness?

What if you could start living a life in which IBS is not an obstacle that keeps you from moving in your chosen direction? What if living your values involves bringing your IBS experiences along for the ride instead of trying to fight them or waiting for them to go away? Can you imagine what that would be like? What if there was something you could do that would enable you to have this vital and full life that you aim for and that you explored in Chapter 4? What if this action exists and is within arm's reach?

Well, there *is* something you can do, and it is called 'acceptance' or 'willingness'. In context of this book we take acceptance to mean making an active choice to take in all the experiences, and willingness to mean being willing and making a conscious choice — hence we use the two terms interchangeably.

Acceptance is the opposite action of avoidance — it is when you willingly make the choice to actively engage your experiences (positive or negative) in a fully embracing manner in the service of living a more vital and valued life. In this context it means to respond to your feelings by actually feeling them, no matter how unpleasant they are, instead of trying to run away from or change them. It also involves actively having and holding your thoughts, like a delicate flower, no matter how distressing or scary they may be. It is embracing the bodily sensations that come along, sensing them fully while adopting a gentle posture towards yourself, contemplating them dispassionately as any other part of your experience. It is also to take in *all* your history or memories, without judgement.

It is important to note that acceptance or willingness is not about taking in your experiences so that you can feel *better*. It is really about *feeling* these experiences better, even the negative ones, in the moment while moving towards your values.

The goal when you accept is to increase your flexibility of responses, or increase your choices. When you are able to accept, or be willing to have those difficult experiences that are out of your control (bodily sensations, emotions, thoughts) in the here and now, without trying to push them away, you also have more awareness of all the other choices you can make. If you are willing to have a bodily sensation, emotion or thought without trying to control it, then the control agenda is undermined as well as all the suffering of a life not lived that comes with it.

If we asked you, 'Do you want a course of injections that will make you feel weak and tired for several months, make all your hair fall out, and make you vomit repeatedly?' You would probably say, 'No, thank you!'

But if you had cancer and this course of injections would totally cure it, you would probably willingly accept to take it without giving too much thought about the side effects. So why would you be willing to put yourself through that? Not because you like, want or approve it, but because you want to do something you value: live. Ultimately this is what acceptance/willingness is all about: making space for the negative symptoms, thoughts and feelings so that you can create a valued life.

At this point go back to the 'What have I been avoiding' exercise in Chapter 3. This will give you a good idea of what it is that you might have to make room for.

Why should you be willing to accept?

In a nutshell: why not? You've tried everything else! You have already been down the road of logical steps. You have tried to analyse your problem, you have tried to change it, control it, eliminate it and numb yourself from it, and the results have not been so good. So why not give acceptance/willingness a chance? What have you got to lose? If it works you will be able to get back on the life track you had planned before IBS came along. If not, at least you gave it a shot and the worst that could happen is for you to end up in the same place you are now.

The ultimate reason for accepting comes from the analysis you made in Chapter 4 of how successfully you are living your values. You have already looked at how trying to fight IBS has stopped or diverted you from living your values. It is like you were climbing your mountain, guided by your values, following a path that made you feel vital and fulfilled. And all of a sudden, this IBS beast appears in your way, with its scary fangs coming out of its wide drooling mouth and enormous claws that threaten to hurt you. You were having such a nice climb and now you see yourself having to fight or run away from this beast. And every time you do this you just see your values going further and further away from you.

But what would happen if you invited the IBS beast to come along with you? Actually, what if you just invited the IBS monster to dinner?

One way to illustrate this is to look at the Uncle Jack metaphor.

Uncle Jack

Imagine that it is your wedding day. You have invited all your extended family for this special occasion; the day is beautiful and you have personally seen to every detail of this celebration so that everyone can enjoy themselves. As your guests arrive you see your mother and father, Aunt Julia who has always been one of your favourites, even Cousin Irving who has been away in Africa for so many years has come to share this special moment in your life. Everyone seems to be enjoying themselves and you feel happy with the way everything is turning out. You are eagerly anticipating the ceremony and hope it runs smoothly.

Then, when you least expect it, you hear a loud blast from an exhaust pipe, and a cloud of smoke invades the area where your celebration will be held. 'It's Uncle Jack!' you immediately think. Uncle Jack is a bit of a character: he can sometimes be a very pleasant and funny man, and some would even say that he can be the life of the party. You have known him all your life and he has been a great support to you at times, so it was very important to you that he comes to your wedding. But lately, Uncle Jack has taken to drinking too much. Sometimes he is able to keep it under control, but most often he is loud, obnoxious and rude to anyone around him and seems to enjoy embarrassing you when he is drunk. But because he is part of the family, you decided to invite him anyway, hoping that he would behave himself.

But today he seems to be at his all-time worst: stumbling between the tables knocking things around, interrupting conversations with offensive remarks and telling embarrassing stories about you. You couldn't think of a worse thing to happen on your wedding day.

Initially you try to limit him to certain areas of the party. You pin him down by the bar since he likes it so much and you ask him to just sit there quietly during the ceremony and then for the rest of the party. He sits quietly for a while, but before you know it he is at it again. This proves to be too much for you and you start shouting, telling him how much you hate him and how you want him to leave. You push him away but he doesn't budge or seem to care about you. He's there for the party and he doesn't intend to go away. You end up letting him stay and try to numb yourself to his presence, but you can't really do it.

As the marriage ceremony approaches your focus gets more and more diverted to trying to keep Uncle Jack under control, but you realise this is impossible. You decide to ask everyone to go home and you postpone your wedding to another date. As people leave you can't take it anymore and you start crying and blaming Uncle Jack for ruining your special occasion. He turns to you and says, 'The invitation you sent me said I would be welcome,' and you respond, 'Yes, but I thought you would have the decency to not show up or at least to have cleaned up your act for today.' Uncle Jack laughs and with a smirk on his face tells you, 'I've always been like this and I will always be like this. And I have no intention of missing your wedding or any other special occasion you might have in the future. In fact I might just drop in at your doorstep at any time I want.'

As Uncle Jack speaks you suddenly realise that you have spent the whole day trying to control or get rid of him and you paid little attention to your guests. You also realise that you ended up missing the most important moment of that day: getting married.

You try to talk to Uncle Jack to see what would be the best possible option from now on:

1 You can try to convince Uncle Jack that if he wants to attend your special occasions, he will have to be on his best behaviour.

2 You can try to numb yourself and essentially remove yourself from your own wedding while Uncle Jack puts on his show.

3 You can avoid your Uncle Jack by never getting married.

4 You can accept Uncle Jack fully, as he is, with all his nasty and unpleasant attributes and enjoy your wedding.

Which of the alternatives do you choose?

Looking through the alternatives, the first one seems quite appealing. If Uncle Jack behaves, everything will be okay. But deep down you know that is not likely to happen, and he has told you that that is the way he is and that he is unlikely to change. Even if it seemed possible you would probably spend your whole wedding day monitoring his behaviour or trying to anticipate what he will do next. Your mind would be so focused on what Uncle Jack was doing (or not) that you wouldn't be able to bring your full attention to one of the most important moments of your life. Now that doesn't seem like a very good wedding day.

What if you could numb or shut yourself out to everything that is going on in your wedding, by drinking or just not interacting with anyone? Although you would still go ahead with the ceremony, how would that make you feel? Would you be able to enjoy it fully? Probably not. In fact, it would be like a big part of you was not attending the wedding at all. What if it wasn't just your wedding? What if it was other situations in your life in which Jack appeared? By numbing yourself how much of a life would you actually be having?

Avoiding Uncle Jack by never getting married doesn't seem much of a solution. It just means that you will never allow yourself to experience the events that you want so much; there will never be a good time to do it as long as Uncle Jack is around. Isn't that missing out on life as well? And how effective will it actually be in keeping Jack away? Didn't he say that he was coming back whenever he wanted, wedding or not?

So, perhaps the only way to have your wedding and truly be present at it — enjoying it for what it means not what it looks like — would involve being willing to have Uncle Jack there as he is. This doesn't mean that you have to approve, like or want Jack and his behaviours, but if it allowed you to move in the direction you most wanted, would you be willing to have him there with you? Trying to control/avoid/eliminate Uncle Jack from the equation doesn't solve the problem and it just keeps you from either getting married or enjoying the ceremony. By being willing to have Uncle Jack with all the unpleasant sensations he causes you, you have time to enjoy your wedding.

This is the essence of acceptance: living with what you cannot control, even if it is unpleasant, and thus actively pursuing the life you want.

Why switch on acceptance?

Acceptance is so important because it allows you to live a vital, engaged and meaningful life every moment. When you accept that you can't get rid of your IBS, you open up space to focus all your energies on pursuing activities that you value. Much like accepting that Uncle Jack is going to be there on your special occasions and will show up from time to time unexpectedly, you don't have to spend your energy trying to control him anymore and you can actually enjoy your wedding.

So far your experience has told you that there are aspects of your life related to your IBS that cannot be changed. Go back to Chapter 3 and check your 'What is avoidance costing you?' exercise. How many times have you let this IBS beast stop you on your way up the mountain? How many times did you try to fight it? How many times did experiential avoidance work in the long term?

It is like having a radio with two switches: the first one controls your IBS and its experiences, and the second one controls your willingness to accept these experiences.

The tricky bit is that you have no real control over the IBS switch. In fact, your experience has shown you that no matter how much you try to control it, it still keeps turning itself on. Sometimes you are able to switch it off for a moment but then it springs back on. Sometimes it looks like it is off but you can still feel it on. Sometimes you choose to ignore it and it turns itself on anyway. In any case, no matter what you do, your IBS switch does its own thing.

But you also have the other switch, the willingness switch. Whether you are willing to accept your IBS is entirely up to you. You have real control over this switch. It is up to you to choose whether you want it off, and with that comes a life of struggle, or if you want it on, in which case you will be able to focus on the more important things in life.

This is something you might have already experienced in the previous chapter with some of the mindfulness exercises. For example, when you choose to sit with your discomfort you are turning on your willingness switch and letting your discomfort switch run its own course. Your discomfort might stay or it might leave but at least you don't get entangled trying to control it. You invite the monsters that you have no control over (discomfort, IBS, Uncle Jack) to come along with you for the ride, which means you can carry on moving in your valued direction no matter what happens.

What acceptance/willingness is not

Being willing is not easy — not because it involves a lot of effort but because it is tricky. Being willing is something that we human beings can learn but it poses a great challenge to our minds. Accepting our bodily sensations, emotions and thoughts in a non-judgemental way in the present moment is a concept that might lead to several misinterpretations, whether because our society has imposed a certain meaning on the word 'acceptance' or because it is difficult not to listen to the judgements and rules that our minds keep creating. With this in mind, we will now make clear what 'acceptance' is *not*.

Acceptance/willingness is not giving up or tolerating

Many people see in the word acceptance a sense of giving up or of having to tolerate something they don't like. When you give up or tolerate you do stop fighting, but in a way you are still involved in the battle. By giving up or tolerating you are taking the losing side of the battle, you are making a deal with your experiences of the if-you-can't-beat-them-join-them sort. The grudge, the hostility and the desire to eliminate the other side are still there, so although the battle is not on the open field, it still rages on. If you feel that acceptance means you have been defeated, you are still in the battle. If you feel that acceptance is about stopping moving forward so that the other side doesn't attack, you are still in the battle. Although this gives you a feeling of things being okay, you are actually sacrificing moving in the direction you want for the sake of not having the war continue. You get trapped in a standstill.

This is quite contrary to what we propose. Acceptance is about stepping aside and seeing the battle play out before you, seeing this battle as a part of your experience and fully embracing both battling sides. Being willing to have this battle going on without being drawn into it means that you don't have to choose a winning or losing side. And that is what acceptance is all about. It is a choice: the choice of moving in your valued direction while willingly having this battle play between your IBS and yourself without having to be a winner or a loser.

Acceptance/willingness is not wanting

If we asked you if you wanted to have all your IBS experiences, odds are that you would respond with a resounding, 'No!' But you notice that we are not asking you to *want* to have the experiences, we are asking you if you *are willing* to have them. There are a lot of things in life that we don't want to do but that we may be willing to do. Someone who goes to the gym regularly surely doesn't want the pain, the exhaustion or the fatigue that exercise gives them, but they are willing to have those experiences in the service of something valued, such as good physical condition. Similarly, you might not want to get up early in the morning to take your kids to school, but if you value your children's education you will probably be willing to do it.

So, being willing to have your IBS experiences doesn't mean that you necessarily like them or want them.

Acceptance/willingness doesn't exclude other strategies

As we said previously, acceptance/willingness is about promoting flexibility of responses. If you already have some strategies that work for you in terms of enabling you to have a more fulfilling life, than by all means we encourage you to keep and make use of them. Some of these might target your symptoms (such as medication or diet) and some might target the associated distress (such as forms of relaxation). As long as these strategies are put in the service of allowing you to live according to your values, they are consistent with what we propose. We suggest that acceptance could be more useful in those situations in which the strategies you use are in the service of eliminating/controlling/avoiding your experiences and not in the service of living your values.

Acceptance/willingness is not trying

When confronted with the possibility of acceptance, some people take a stance of, 'Okay, I guess I'll try to be more willing to accept my difficult experiences.' This is a common pitfall of willingness. Willingness is a choice — you either do it or you don't. When you 'try' you are actually not fully engaging with the situation. It is like you approach the situation in the perspective of, 'I would like to be willing ... but it's pretty scary, so I'll just try.' And suddenly you are back in a web of entanglement with your thoughts as your mind tells you what you can and can't do, and what you 'should' do. You can limit the where, when or how long you are willing to accept, but what you can't limit is how much you accept.

There are many things in our experience that we cannot 'try'. For example, try to close your eyes. Don't actually close them, just try to close them. This is impossible to do, because you will always have your eyes either closed or open, but there is no way you can 'try' to close them. Acceptance is much like this; you either follow your choice to accept or you don't.

Acceptance is a movement like jumping; you can decide whether you jump from a chair, a desk, a window or an airplane, but once you choose to jump, that is it, you just jump, you don't try to jump.

Acceptance/willingness is not conditional

This brings us back to the on/off characteristic of willingness. What we mean by it not being conditional is that when you turn it on you can't do it on the basis of, 'I'll turn it on, but when it starts to feel too difficult I'll turn it off.' When you apply these conditions to your willingness — conditions that depend on the quality of the experience — you are not truly embracing your experiences. You can, however, limit willingness. You can assign a time, place or situation limit, for which you will be willing to accept difficult experiences. Such as, 'I am willing to go to the shop for five minutes with my difficult IBS experiences, but not for thirty minutes.'

Choosing to accept

As we have said, you might have had a glimpse of acceptance in some of the exercises of the previous chapters, but acceptance is not a matter of chance. It is an active and conscious choice. Remember what we said before about the two switches you have in your life. What if to live the life you really want and value, you have to consciously reach out and turn your willingness switch on? Are you willing, in this present moment, to have your IBS experiences fully and without defence, as they are, not as your mind says they are, looking at them from your observer perspective so that you can pursue your chosen life values?

This is a yes-or-no answer; there is no middle ground. As we said before, willingness is like jumping: you are either jumping or you are not.

If your answer is no, think about why you answered this way. Try to see what reasons your mind came up with for you to give that answer. Revise what not accepting is costing you. Try to think of the valued path you could achieve by choosing to turn your willingness switch on. If it is still too hard to come to a yes answer, maybe working with defusion and mindfulness for a while longer will help you see a way that you can embrace your IBS experiences.

If by the time you were finishing the question you were already answering yes; if you did so without thinking, you are probably ready to start working on acceptance. The following exercises in this chapter are designed to help you do just that.

Do you have your tools?

Before starting to put your acceptance into practice, it is useful to have a quick look at the important tools you already have and those you have been developing to help with your willingness.

There is a reason we guided you first through the defusion and mindfulness exercises. One of the key elements in acceptance is to start it from the observing-self point in the here and now. Using mindfulness techniques, you will be able to contact this sense of self and bring your attention and focus to what is happening in the present moment.

Also, because it is something new and illogical, your mind is bound to react to what you are doing. If your mind starts predicting awful consequences or giving you arguments about how IBS really needs to be eliminated first, try to notice those thoughts and recognise them for what they are — just thoughts. In situations like this, try to notice what your experience of following these thoughts tells you: is doing what your mind says going to work?

Now, if you are willing, let's begin to put acceptance into practice.

Exercise: Turning the acceptance switch on

In this exercise we will ask you to turn your willingness switch on for some minutes, as in the radio metaphor. To do this, first you need to find a suitable situation in which to practise your acceptance.

Think of an action or goal that is consistent with your values but that you are not comfortable with at this moment. Looking at the values-consistent goals you wrote down in Chapter 4 might help with this. It doesn't have to be something you feel is impossible for you now, it might actually be something that you are already doing but that carries a level of discomfort that normally you try to avoid or get rid of. What we are trying to find here is essentially a goal that is both small enough for you to handle as a first approach and at the same time is challenging enough to bring up the experiences you have been struggling with.

Write down a situation that you think might have these characteristics:

_____

_____

_____

_____

Once you have a situation in your mind make sure you are clear about what you are committing to accept. Remember, you will not be merely _trying_ to accept, and once you choose to accept you cannot make it dependent on how uncomfortable the situation feels. Set yourself the limits that you can control such as place, time, quantifiable small goals (for example, if you are taking a bus ride it could be the number of stops you are willing to ride for).

Now that you have everything ready you will be faced with the choice of turning your acceptance switch on or leaving it off. Your mind will probably do its best to try and keep it off. Maybe it is time to step into your observer-self position and use some defusion techniques.

It is time then to turn it on and for the duration you have set just embrace all your difficult IBS experiences, taking them with you, while you move in the direction of your valued goal.

With practice you will be able to turn the switch on for longer or to do it in more difficult situations.

If you have doubts, check below when Angela first switched her willingness on.

When Angela first undertook this exercise, she found it hard to get the right balance between manageability and challenge. Initially she came up with the goal of returning to her classes. Although this was a values-consistent goal and a very important one for her, it was also a very difficult one to take as a first step since it was one of the situations she avoided the most. As you might remember, growth and learning was one of the most important values for Angela. Working with this value in mind Angela found that there were other situations related to this value that were more manageable, such as reading something related to her degree for thirty minutes every day. This was a challenging task for her because it brought up memories of the incidents she had in class, and the feelings of embarrassment and sadness for having left her degree. But still, Angela picked up her book every day, knowing that she would have to make room for all these difficult experiences. Her mind kept telling her not to do it, that it would be a waste of time. When faced with these thoughts Angela made room for them and kept her willingness switch on. By choosing to do this over, for instance, watching TV to numb herself to these difficult experiences, Angela had an opportunity to watch her uncomfortable thoughts and feelings while doing something that was values consistent. This was only the first step for Angela, and a very important one. From this step she was able to develop her acceptance/willingness skills and use them over and over again in many other different steps that she wanted to take. Every step she took brought her difficult experiences that she made room for in order to keep moving in her valued direction. After many of these steps Angela resumed her degree.

Exercise: What is the shape of your IBS beast?

IBS is one of the many parts of your experience, but because it is intertwined with your body and mind it is sometimes hard to see what it is that needs to be accepted. One way to do this is to give IBS a shape by imagining how it would look if it were standing in front of you.

In order to achieve this you will have to consciously come into contact with your IBS experiences. Think, for instance, of a particular time of the day that this is likely to happen (your fusion diary might be helpful here). See if you can mindfully contact your IBS experience and just observe it. Now try to focus on your IBS bodily sensations and imagine how these would look like if they were outside your body. Close your eyes and try to picture it as you answer the following questions.

If your IBS bodily sensation were in front of you, what shape would it be?

_____

_____

_____

_____

If your IBS bodily sensation were in front of you, how big would it be?

_____

_____

_____

_____

If your IBS bodily sensation were in front of you, what colour would it be?

_____

_____

_____

_____

If your IBS bodily sensation were in front of you, how powerful would it be?

_____

_____

_____

If your IBS bodily sensation had a speed, how fast would it go?

_____

_____

_____

If your IBS bodily sensation were in front of you, what sort of texture would it have (smooth, porous, rough, etc.)?

_____

_____

_____

If your IBS bodily sensation had an aroma, how would it smell?

_____

_____

_____

If your IBS bodily sensation had a weight, how much would it weigh?

_____

_____

_____

If your IBS bodily sensation had a voice, how would it sound?

_____

_____

_____

Once you have this image of your IBS bodily sensation in front of you, what response does this bring? Does it come with any difficult thoughts or feelings attached to it? If it does, try to give them a shape as well. You can use the same questions as a guide. You will probably end up with two or more of these beasts in front of you.

Now that they are there, staring you in the face, see if you can stretch your arm out and touch them. Can you have them as they are, not as they say they are?

Now it is time to welcome them back where they belong: inside you. In your mind's eye wrap your arms around them and embrace them back into your body. Remember this is where they live, and they need to be allowed to live there. Show these monsters the same compassion you would show yourself if you were lost and hurt. After all, they are a part of your experience.

Exercise: Looking for belly discomfort

What we would like you to do now is to get into your observing-self seat and actually go out and try to find your belly discomfort (bodily sensations associated with IBS). Whether or not it shows up is not the point; the important thing is to be willing to have it there.

Start by sitting down and closing your eyes. Focus on your breathing until you can feel yourself being in the observing-self seat. Once you are looking from your observing self, scan your body from head to toe to see if you can find any sort of discomfort. If something stands out, just focus on it and try to feel its energy flow. See if you can make room for that uncomfortable energy, you can even rub your hand in the place where it is feeling uncomfortable, as if you were petting your discomfort. Just open yourself to it and observe yourself welcoming it.

Now focus on your belly. Try to feel all the parts of it — the parts that are in contact with your clothes; the tightness around your waist from your trousers or skirt. See if you can feel the inside, your muscles underneath your skin, your stomach, your liver. See if you can feel the movements that occur in your belly to push the food along its way. Now think of how important your belly is for you, how essential it is for your survival. Think also of all the important occasions in life that are marked by a meal and how that relates to your belly. If this brings up any discomfort or any thoughts or feelings related to your belly, see if you can just make room for them; be compassionate towards yourself and towards this experience. If you feel any type of discomfort just allow yourself to have it.

Now scan your body again and see if there are other areas of discomfort. As you take notice of every other part of your body, do it compassionately and allow yourself to feel them completely. If more thoughts or feelings come along, make space for them as well.

Bring yourself back into the room and jot down on a card all the difficult bodily sensations, thoughts and feelings that came along while you did this exercise. Carry that card with you for the next week in your wallet, purse or pocket. This symbolises your ability to willingly carry something that you don't necessarily want with you, while you engage in other activities.

You can do this as many times as you like, and you will probably see that you can carry a lot more than you give yourself credit for. Just notice what the experience is like when you find the card from time to time.

Exercise: Accepting every day

Each day presents plenty of opportunities to practise your acceptance skills. During the next week try to approach your difficult IBS situations using acceptance. What we are asking you to do is engage in activities that are meaningful and valued for you even if they bring up IBS distress — but we would like you to approach these situations from the perspective of your observing self, making room for your IBS.

Undertaking this exercise over the period of a week will give you a fair chance to evaluate how acceptance works for you. We hope that approaching valued situations with acceptance will get you closer to the valued life you want to live.

Are you willing to have IBS?

A good way to approach this is to come up with a list of these situations. Try to think of situations that are likely to come up this week that have been a challenge for you in the past because of the physical or mental discomfort they provoke; write these in the first column of table below. In the second column, rate how challenging these situations are for you: 10 would be extremely challenging and 1 would be hardly challenging. After you have jotted them down, go out and try them on with your acceptance, mindfulness and defusion skills.

Situation	Challenge level
1.	
2.	
3.	
4.	
5.	
6.	
7.	
8.	
9.	
10.	

Check Angela's list of difficult situations if you need a little help.

Situation	Challenge level
1. Going out to do the shopping	7
2. Any of my meals	5
3. Going out to meet my friends	9
4. Going out for exercise	8
5. Taking the bus to go anywhere	8
6. Explaining to my parents what is happening to me	5
7. Thinking of going back to classes	8
8. Reading books or anything related to my degree	6
9. Doing the house chores	4
10. Going to the park and watching other people be carefree	4

Once you have your list, the goal is to actively pursue these situations with mindfulness and acceptance. Some activities might be more difficult than others, so you can start by having a go at the ones you consider less challenging and build your acceptance skills from there.

Starting out with small steps is not an excuse to not address the big ones. Once you truly own your skills, go for the hardest ones, the 8s, 9s and 10s.

It is likely that these situations will be the most difficult to address, but they are also probably linked to some of your more important values, so the potential to get closer to your valued life is also greater.

Remember also that you are not limited to the situations you listed in the table. Every moment might present itself as an opportunity to practise acceptance, and it is up to you to take notice of that moment and choose acceptance.

You might like to keep track of your progress with this exercise. Once you have faced your difficult situation, spend some time reflecting on the event and answer the following questions. Whether you photocopy this page or you keep your own journal, have a go at these questions once you have exercised your acceptance in your difficult situations. (You will also find extra copies in the appendix of this book.)

What was the situation?

_____

_____

_____

_____

What difficult experiences came up before and during your engagement with this situation (such as bodily sensations, feelings, thoughts)?

_____

_____

_____

_____

What was your mind telling you about all this?

_____

_____

_____

_____

What skills (defusion, mindfulness or others) did you use to accept the situation? How did they work?

_____

_____

_____

_____

Could you improve the use of these skills in the future to be more successful in your acceptance? If yes, how?

_____

_____

_____

_____

_____

Living the life you want

By the end of this chapter you have probably already been involved in situations in which by choosing to accept the difficult content you had a taste of how this allowed you to move in a valued direction.

Now that you have the skills to start approaching your valued life again, it is time to make a plan and commit to it. To find out how to do this, read on.

CHAPTER 8

Committing to make your own music

Imagine that you are the conductor of an orchestra, and that you have been conducting the symphony of your life. As in any orchestra you have several musicians coming in to contribute the sound of their instruments. These musicians represent your memories, bodily sensations, thoughts and emotions. Some of the musicians who show up to play are lovely, accomplished musicians capable of producing amazing music, and they are very keen to be conducted by you. They are musicians capable of together playing tunes such as 'That wonderful picnic you had with someone special in the park' or 'That lovely meal you had for your best friend's birthday at their place three years ago' or even 'That feeling of accomplishment you have once you finish one of your work objectives with great results'. You really hope that these musicians will be in the front rows of the orchestra so you can appreciate their great work from your conductor's stand.

But some other musicians you really don't like have appeared as well. They look frightening, they really don't even know how to play and their only purpose is to make as much noise as they can. Among these musicians are most of your IBS beasts, including the ones you met in the previous chapter. These musicians are called 'pain', 'bowel discomfort' or 'embarrassment' and all they want is to play music such as 'Stay at home' or 'Be afraid of what we can do to you' or 'You will always feel unwell, so you might as well give up'.

After a while these unruly musicians start coming to the front of the orchestra pit, pushing away all the musicians you like to the back rows. So whenever you try to get your orchestra to play, although you can hear your favourite musicians in the background playing the lovely music you want, all that stands out to you is the noise that these beastly musicians sitting in the front rows are creating. Soon these beasts start shouting, telling you what sort of music you should be playing and threatening to make even more noise if you don't get the orchestra to play what they want.

Sometimes you argue with these musicians and try to get them to leave the concert hall so that you can work with the musicians you really like. But these musicians refuse to leave, and it seems that every time you try to push them out the door they either make even more noise or they leave for a while and come back bigger and noisier than before. You have probably been involved in this struggle with your IBS experiences several times before, spending a good deal of your time trying to argue with or get rid of these nasty musicians.

But let's consider what happened while you were fighting and arguing with these unruly music players. The music stopped. The first thing you had to do was to put your 'life symphony' on hold so that you could direct your efforts to getting the musicians out of the concert hall. Did these guys leave? Probably not!

You try to play that beautiful flute part that is called 'Sitting in a café and relaxing by reading the newspaper' but the noisy trumpet musicians of pain and bowel discomfort keep blowing the 'Stay at home' song louder and louder as they push their way closer and closer to the front of the orchestra pit. When you realise that they are there to stay and that they are going to keep trying to take over the front rows so that they have your full attention, you decide to try to negotiate with them. You say, 'Okay, I'll play what you want me to play but just go to the back of the orchestra pit so I don't have to listen to your noise too much.' You also make a deal with yourself saying, 'Maybe I can get used to this kind of brassy and drummy music' or 'Maybe I won't miss my lovely flutes so much.'

As time passes you keep playing this music that has nothing to do with what you really wanted in the first place. And every time you try to conduct the orchestra towards playing the music you like, those beastly musicians stand up and start coming to the front again or they just make more noise than usual in the back to remind you of what they are capable — and you go back to try to appease them by playing their choice of music.

And it doesn't stop here, because when you play the music these beasts want you to play, some other musicians outside the concert hall hear it and decide to invite themselves to the concert as well. So all of a sudden you have musicians called 'regret', 'hopelessness', 'shame', 'embarrassment', 'anxiety' or 'anger', just to name a few, coming in to make some noise as well.

Now imagine that one day you wake up and slowly it dawns on you that you are still the conductor of the orchestra, and that as conductor it is actually up to *you* to choose which music will be played that day. You realise that no matter how much those IBS beasts snarl, growl and threaten you to play their music, the decision is *yours*.

So you go out and choose to play your 'I am going to see my friend for coffee' tune. This is a very important piece of music for you because it always makes you feel alive and vibrant. Immediately your IBS beasts get up and start shouting, 'You better go back home or we'll blow these horns so loud that you'll have bowel pain for hours. Now just go back to playing the "Being at home feeling sorry for myself" music!' Although you hear what they say and you start to hear the horns, you keep conducting the whole orchestra to play the music you want, without bothering to try to fight, argue or kick out the beasts. What do you think will happen? Maybe the beasts get closer and shout even louder, maybe they even blow a horn or two. Again you hear and feel what these beasts are saying but you choose to keep playing your music by going out and meeting your friend. And this is just one example of the several choices you can make; you might want to play the 'I am going to exercise', the 'I will go on holiday', the 'I will go to work' or the 'I will do my daily chores' music or any other tune that is truly meaningful to you.

The following day, as you come in to the concert hall you see your IBS beasts angry and trying to look more threatening than ever, but still you come in and start to conduct one of your favourite songs. Although they try to disrupt you, you continue to conduct the music you chose for that day.

And so it continues for the following days, weeks, months. With the power of choice in your hands you play the music that fills you with a sense of vitality instead of the music your IBS beasts demand you play. You don't argue or try to kick out the beasts. You recognise them as being there and you continue to conduct the music *you* chose. Much like in the Uncle Jack example, you invite your beasts to stay and you make it clear that no matter how much they threaten you, the music being played will be of your choice.

Can you imagine this happening? What do you think will happen to your beastly musicians in time? What would it mean to you to play *your* choice of life symphony, even if some notes might sound a bit off in the middle? What would that be like?

Committed action

So far in this book you have learned the skills that allow you to have difficult thoughts, bodily sensations, feelings and memories, by making room for them so that you can live your life the way you most value. By opening up to your IBS experiences you have made a conscious choice to be willing to have them so that trying to control/avoid/eliminate them will not stand in the way of pursuing your vital ambitions.

By using this book and the acceptance, defusion and mindfulness skills you have learned, you might have caught a glimpse of that wonderful music you really want to hear. But this is not all. Having a new perspective is very useful and it might even turn your world upside down for a while, but something else is needed so that you can play your symphony every day. What is needed is committed action.

When you commit to be truly willing to accept your difficult experiences, you gain a real control of the music that is being played in your life. Being able to accept is very good, but you need to translate that into committed actions that move you in your valued directions. To put it simply, you have to decide where you want to go, make a plan to go in that direction and then actually go.

Remember: being willing is not about biting your lip and pushing through the difficult experiences that IBS brings you. When you combine committed action with willingness you are climbing back on your conductor's stand and directing your symphony no matter how much the 'bad' musicians protest. So what will you do with those musicians? Try to ignore them? Try to make them leave? You've tried these approaches. Is it possible to make your own music, made up of all the parts in it that you love *and* a few parts that you don't like? Is it possible for you to use all the techniques you have been working at, such as mindfulness and defusion, so that you can take what all the musicians are offering you and still conduct the symphony of your life?

Reasons

Committed action might sound very simple, but again, it is tricky. When you commit, it is likely that your mind is going to start looking for 'reasons' to do so. And because it is your mind it will probably come up with many 'reasons' why you should not commit as well.

First of all, it is important to distinguish reasons from facts. For example, take the reason: 'I can't go to work because I am too tired.' Does being 'too tired' make it physically impossible to go to work? No. You can feel tired and still go. Many people go to work while feeling tired and are still able to perform to a high standard. We could just as easily have used a more positive reason, such as: 'I will go to work because I'm feeling full of energy today.' Again, does feeling you have a lot of energy make any difference to being able to go to work? Not really. If people only went to work when they are feeling very energetic there wouldn't be much work done. So being 'too tired' or 'full of energy' are just reasons and not facts that might influence your decision to go to work. A fact could be something such as: 'I can't go to work because there is 6 feet of snow blocking the entrance of my house and all the roads are closed.' *That* would be a fact.

But why is it so important to talk about reasons? Because reasons can influence your choices. If you choose to follow your values based on reasons then you set yourself up to see your values pursuit change according to changes in your reasons. So in the previous example you would condition your choice of going to work to whatever reason was stronger that day, and you would stay in if you were tired or go to work if you felt energetic.

Committed action is all about choices, but these choices are not dictated by reasons. You can *choose* to follow the skills you learned in this book because they made sense to you, but you can also *choose* not to. You can *choose* to go out and exercise even if you are in pain, but you can also *choose* not to.

What if making your choice doesn't depend on reasons? What if choosing to move in a certain direction is independent of whatever reasons come up to support or attack that move? What would determine the choices you make?

Remember your values?

Yes — your values determine the choices you make. Remember when you explored your values in Chapter 4? The values you identified came from a place where there are no reasons. For instance, people don't value being good parents because of reasons; they just know they want to be good parents. If you ask them repeatedly why they value this, they might try to come up with some reasons, such as, 'It's the proper thing to do,' or 'Because my children need me.' But don't you think they would still value these even if society told them that being a good parent is not proper? Don't parents still value being good parents even when their children have no needs and are a long way from home with their own children? If you kept asking them why they value being good parents, eventually they would probably just run out of reasons and tell you, 'I just value that for no reason at all.' So even if they ran out of reasons they would still value being good parents.

This is why we spent so much time and took such care in exploring your values back in Chapter 4: because when it comes to committed action, it is your values that will point your way. To move in your valued direction you have to make the choice of moving in that direction despite any reasons that might come along. When you move in your valued direction there are no good or bad reasons to do it, because the end result will always be the same: feeling more vital and full.

Before moving on to the exercise that follows, take a moment to revisit your values and your valued actions in Chapter 4. If you feel that by reading the chapters that followed those exercises you would word your values or your valued goals in a different way, try to rephrase them in the light of how you understand them now.

Exercise: Making a commitment plan

It is now time to take everything you have learned in this book and put it into practice. As we said before, although making a commitment seems quite easy, there are some tricky bits to it. In order to help you build a committed action we have broken this process into several parts: confirming your direction, taking action, making room, taking the last step and sticking to your chosen value.

Confirming your direction

Start out by being sure of the direction you want to take. For that you have to consult your values. You can do this exercise for just one value at a time, though you will need to repeat it for each value. Maybe for the first one, choose a value that you have neglected for some time or that you have lost touch with (the Zorg exercise in Chapter 4 may be helpful in identifying such a value). Now jot it down.

The value I want to pursue is:

_____

Taking action

When deciding how to take action that is consistent with the value you just chose to pursue, it is helpful first to look at what you have been doing that is inconsistent with that value and how much it costs you.

What I have been doing that is inconsistent with my value is:

_____

This has cost me (for example, relationships, health, time, money, distress):

_____

Now think of what it is that you want to do that is consistent with your value. A goal that is both achievable and challenging would be a great way to start. Check the goals you set out for this value in Chapter 4. If the goals you chose are too difficult at this point, see if you can break them down into achievable parts that would still be consistent with your values and that would eventually lead you to achieve the larger goal. You can think of this a bit like having to cross a shallow river on your journey east: although you might not be able to jump across in one go, you could put a stepping stone in from the bank you are standing on; then from that stepping stone you could put down another stepping stone, and another and another. So, what are the stepping stones involved in crossing this river that will enable you to keep travelling east?

The goal I want to achieve is:

_____

_____

Now try to be specific in terms of what actions you are going to take to achieve this goal. Think of the day, the time, the place in which you are going to do it. Think for how long or in what situation you will carry out these actions. Describe every action that is going to be undertaken and the order in which they will follow.

I commit to take the following actions in the following circumstances:

_____

_____

_____

_____

_____

Making room

Finally, think of all the things you are going to have to make room for while pursuing this valued action. Think what you will have to be willing to accept or allow to be present.

In order to perform my valued action I am willing to make room for the following *sensations in my body*:

_____

_____

_____

_____

In order to perform my valued action I am willing to make room for the following *thoughts or images*:

_____

_____

_____

_____

In order to perform my valued action I am willing to make room for the following *feelings or emotions*:

_____

_____

_____

_____

In order to perform my valued action I am willing to make room for the following *urges to avoid*:

_____

_____

_____

_____

Taking the last step

You have jotted down where you want to go, how and when you want to move in that direction, and the sensations, thoughts, emotions and urges that you will have to bring along with you. It is now time to go out and do it. The distance between what you have just written down and living a valued life is only one action away, so just do it.

Many people get stuck at this very last step because it feels a bit scary — if this is you, why not invite that fear along for the ride as well? Like we said before, your mind will be buzzing with reasons to do it or not do it. See if, just for a moment, you can notice who is giving you these reasons? This is a good time to step into your observing-self shoes and defuse from all the advice your mind is giving you by recognising these as thoughts and reasons, thanking your mind for them and then continuing to move in the direction you are committed to. We will give you a more structured approach to dealing with barriers in the next chapter, but for now just try to recognise your barriers and see if you can make space to bring them along with you.

Sticking to your chosen value

We would like you to stick with the value you chose for the next week. Depending on the actions you chose to start this journey with, this might mean repeating the same action for a number of days (for example, if you chose exercising for ten minutes every day, or getting on a bus for four stops four days of the week) or coming up with different actions that will amount to a greater goal (for example, if your main goal is to go out for a meal you might choose to break that into several actions that can be spaced throughout the week, including calling a friend or relative to go with you, booking the restaurant, going out for the meal).

Alternatively you might choose to tackle more than one value during the week. If you choose to do so be mindful of how much you can actually achieve and check if this is not just another form of avoidance because sticking to the same value for a whole week is too scary.

To make it easier to plan your week, opposite is a form you can use to complete the exercise you just did (you will find more blank copies in the appendix of this book). Carry these around with you once they are filled in — this will be a symbol of the contract you made with yourself: the contract of life.

Commitment diary

Day: __/__/__

The value I want to pursue is:

_____
_____
_____
_____

What I have been doing that is inconsistent with my value is:

_____
_____
_____
_____

This has cost me (for example, relationships, health, time, money, distress):

_____
_____
_____
_____

The goal I want to achieve is:

_____
_____
_____
_____

I commit to take the following actions in the following circumstances:

_____

_____

_____

_____

In order to perform my valued action I am willing to make room for the following *sensations in my body*:

_____

_____

_____

_____

In order to perform my valued action I am willing to make room for the following *thoughts or images*:

_____

_____

_____

_____

In order to perform my valued action I am willing to make room for the following *feelings or emotions*:

_____

_____

_____

_____

In order to perform my valued action I am willing to make room for the following *urges to avoid* :

_____

_____

_____

_____

If you undertook the previous exercise for a week, you probably saw yourself doing things that you were not doing before. Actions that you previously avoided were put into practice because they have an important meaning to you. And you probably realised that by sticking to those actions you have opened the door to more and more actions that will lead you in the direction you value most. So you started to give yourself more and more choices. The process of committed action is all about shifting from a life constricted by avoidance and fusion to a life where forward movement in the direction of a valued goal and an expansion of your choices and actions is constant. When you are acting and moving in a way that is consistent with your values you will probably experience this sense of expansion in your life. The next exercise might help you to get a feel for that.

Exercise: The bubble

Imagine that your life is a bubble made of a special material that can absorb all things that are around the bubble without ever breaking or bursting it. You are the one controlling how much air goes into the bubble, therefore how much it expands or contracts. Outside the bubble you have sharp objects called your IBS experiences. When you become scared about these sharp objects because they are going to burst your bubble, you stop inflating it and your life contracts. When you accept these experiences into your life despite of how sharp they *look* and you willingly inflate your bubble so that it comes in contact with them and absorbs them, your bubble expands.

Now go back and take a look at the committed actions you undertook last week. See if these actions were done in the service of your values and fully embracing all experiences. We will call these vital actions. See also if there were examples of non-vital actions. These could be actions that you had planned to do but ended up not doing in the service of avoiding your IBS experiences, in the service of reasons, in the service of proving something to yourself or others or even of just not wanting to be beaten. It is okay if some actions felt non-vital; after all, you are still taking your first steps towards your valued life.

In the table below jot down the actions you undertook, and mark with an X whether you think they were vital or non-vital. In the next column mark again with an X whether you felt that this action led you to a sense of expansion in your life or to a sense of contraction.

Action	Vital	Non-vital	Expansion	Contraction

Finally, take a moment to think and jot down some thoughts about what it felt like when you experienced your life expanding and what it felt like when you experienced your life contracting.

Expansion felt like:

_____

_____

_____

Contraction felt like:

_____

_____

_____

Expanding in your chosen directions

Every time you commit to an action that is congruent with your values you add a new action to your repertoire and you are presented with more choices. In other words, you experience expansion in your life. This experience will probably give you confidence to take the next step towards a committed action, and the next and the next …

By committing to your vital actions every day you will be able to further expand your life in the directions you value, even if IBS comes along with it. Expansion will happen continually if you follow your valued path, for this path has no end and there is always more east that you can travel to.

Can you imagine what it would be like to have that feeling of expanding life every day? Can you imagine living the way you want to live no matter what life throws at you? Wouldn't you like to come to your 100th birthday party and look back at a life like that?

Be alive every day!

This book was created to help you live the life you most want to live, instead of spending fruitless energy trying to get rid of IBS. If you have followed the advice in this book and practised the exercises, you have done the core work that will enable you to do this for the rest of your life. You have your tools of defusion, mindfulness and acceptance. You know your values, so you know where you want to go, and you know how to achieve that by committing to that path, maybe using a stepping-stone approach if it is useful. All that is left now is to expand what you have done in this chapter for one value to all the other important values in your life. Most importantly, you need to choose to live by your values every day.

Really living with IBS is choosing to commit to your values every day even when IBS gets in the way. We hope that this book has helped you to choose to be alive every day!

You may come across some barriers on your journey, and as we promised, we will dedicate our final chapter to those barriers and to teach you what you can do when they come up. We hope this will help you stay with your commitments.

CHAPTER 9

Staying committed

In the previous chapter while working through your commitment exercises you may have glimpsed the fullness of a life lived in the service of your values. Maybe you worked on one value consistently or maybe you chose to tackle several of your valued directions. In any case you have made the first and most vital step, the one of actually beginning. As we said in the previous chapter, the challenge is now to expand your commitment to several valued areas of your life, and to do so every day. If you have done that, congratulations! If not, this chapter will help you.

Barriers

Have you felt that putting your valued committed actions into practice is sometimes harder than it initially seemed? Do you find yourself from time to time going back to the same controlling agenda you had before? Are there barriers in your life that seem to force you to go back to those old strategies?

Because human beings are creatures of habit, it is very easy to find yourself slipping back into old patterns whenever barriers appear in your way. Sometimes it might seem that life places impassable walls in the way of your valued path, and you find yourself going back to trying to eliminate, avoid or control the wall in some way — so it is important to know how to address these barriers if they come up.

But before we address ways to deal with barriers, it is important to know how to identify if they are standing in your way. One way to do this is to keep track of how you are living that valued life and how consistent you are being with your committed actions.

Exercise: Are you living in the bullseye?

Take a moment to think about the past week. Below, you will see a dartboard containing all the valued domains you have explored.[1] Now try to think of how you feel you lived according to each of these valued domains in the last week, and mark X in the appropriate spot. The bullseye represents you feeling that you have fully lived your life according to your values in the past week; the circles further away from the bullseye represent feeling that you lived in a manner far away from your value.

1 Far from
2 Not close
3 Close
4 Very close
5 Bullseye

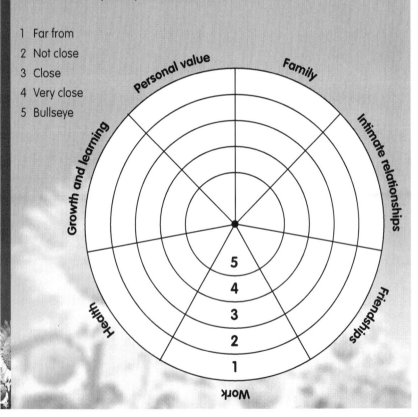

In the next part of this exercise you will see a similar dartboard, but this one refers to how consistent you think your actions were with your values in the past week. Try to think of how often you persisted in undertaking the committed actions relevant to that value even in the face of barriers. The bullseye means that you have always persisted with your committed action even when faced with barriers; the outside ring indicates that you did not persist once you encountered a barrier. Now mark with an X to show how much you believe you persisted in each domain.

1 Did not
2 Persisted at
3 Often
4 Almost always
5 Bullseye (always persisted)

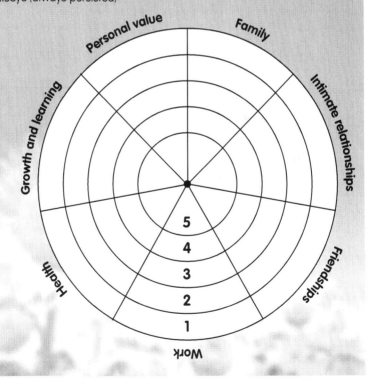

Within this exercise you can find two distinguished purposes. The first part gives you a chance to look back at all your valued domains in life and check if you really feel that you are living them in a full or close-to-full manner. This will point to any areas that you are finding particularly difficult to deal with. The second part of the exercise will give you an idea of not only what barriers are coming up for you, but also of how much these are standing in your way. This will be very valuable for the next exercises.

The combination of the two parts of the exercise might uncover that you are struggling with one of your valued paths because you are not being persistent enough in your actions. This could indicate that you need to revise some of your strategies or that you need to break down your goals into smaller pieces. Another thing you might uncover is that persisting in a particular valued action is not enough to make you feel that you are living in the bullseye. If so, ask yourself if it is time to take on a new challenge in that valued area. Is this area really of value to you? Finally, ask yourself if your mind's tendency to be judgemental is getting in the way of just noticing your progress along your valued path.

Another purpose of this exercise is to allow you to monitor your own progress at any time. This is particularly helpful in the first few weeks after you start to use committed action in the service of your values because it will point out what still needs to be worked on or tweaked. This does not mean, however, that its use stops there. At any point in your life this is a great quick exercise that helps you get a pulse for what is happening in your life.

Revisiting barriers

Barriers come in all shapes and sizes. Although in this book we have focused on the types of barriers that are generated by your IBS, the fact is that life in general is good at placing obstacles in the way of our valued paths. But what can you do when a barrier stands between you and the valued life you want so much?

The answer is simple: you can use the techniques you have developed over the course of this book.

It is easy to run into situations that make your life difficult, in which everything including your IBS will seem too much to bear. You will see mighty stones appear in your path up the mountain, and your mind (as always) will be buzzing with thoughts, plans and reasons that might lead you to engage in a fight with the stone or take a path different from the one you value.

When this happens, and it *will* happen — after all, it is part of this wonderful experience we call living — you will know what to do. You will be able to use your defusion techniques to see your thoughts as they are and not what they say they are. You will be able to sit on the observer seat and look at your barriers from a perspective in which you can hold and carry them with you; you will be able to willingly embrace these barriers and take them along on your valued path. You will know what it has cost you to fight or avoid these obstacles. You will have come to know what it is to really be in touch with what you most want to be about. You will have asked yourself on many occasions: Am I willing to have this obstacle as it is and still do what needs to be done to stay on my valued path?

In the bullseye exercise you might have come across some of the barriers that are keeping you from living that valued life you want so much. Some of them may still be related to your IBS, some may not. In any case, if you are currently facing obstacles, the following exercises will help you.

Exercise: Identifying barriers

Take a moment to think of your valued directions and what is keeping you from moving in that direction at this point. What is the barrier? It could be related to your IBS, but it can also be related to anything that you feel poses a barrier at this point. Is your mind giving you a lot of chatter about how you can't do this or that? Try to catch the thoughts and reasons your mind is giving you not to engage in your committed actions, and jot them down. Look at some of the barriers that Angela's mind was giving her if you need some help.

Barrier 1:

_____

_____

_____

Barrier 2:

_____

_____

_____

Barrier 3:

_____

_____

_____

Barrier 4:

_____

_____

_____

Barrier 5:

_____

_____

_____

Barrier 6:

_____

_____

_____

Barrier 7:

_____

_____

_____

Barrier 8:

_____

_____

_____

Angela's barriers

Barrier 1: You have dropped out of your degree before. What makes you think you will make it now?

Barrier 2: You know you will not last for a whole lecture if it's too long. Are you going to embarrass yourself again by leaving in the middle of it?

Barrier 3: How do you expect to get a job if you don't even have your qualifications yet?

Barrier 4: Why should you be the one making the effort to call your parents? They never call you!

Barrier 5: You have tried eating your five serves of fruit and vegetables each day before and you didn't last more than a week. It's not going to be different this time.

Barrier 6: Why bother trying to get a date; you'll have nothing interesting to say to the other person.

Barrier 7: You can't afford to join a gym, and even if you could you don't have the motivation to go.

Barrier 8: You have isolated yourself from your friends, so why would they want to see you again now?

Exercise: Committed action plans for barriers

As we said before, the techniques you can use to deal with your barriers are pretty much the same as those you have used previously in this book. Go back to your barriers and see if you can accept them and carry them with you on your valued journey. See what techniques you have learned that could help make this happen. See what actions you need to undertake that will enable you to continue on your valued path while carrying these barriers. Again take a look at Angela's example.

What needs to be accepted for barrier 1?

_____

What skills could be useful for barrier 1?

_____

Staying committed

Committed action for barrier 1:

_____

What needs to be accepted for barrier 2?

_____

What skills could be useful for barrier 2?

_____

Committed action for barrier 2:

_____

What needs to be accepted for barrier 3?

_____

What skills could be useful for barrier 3?

_____

Committed action for barrier 3:

_____

What needs to be accepted for barrier 4?

_____

What skills could be useful for barrier 4?

_____

Committed action for barrier 4:

_____

What needs to be accepted for barrier 5?

What skills could be useful for barrier 5?

_____

Committed action for barrier 5:

_____

What needs to be accepted for barrier 6?

_____

What skills could be useful for barrier 6?

_____

Committed action for barrier 6:

_____

What needs to be accepted for barrier 7?

_____

What skills could be useful for barrier 7?

_____

Committed action for barrier 7:

_____

What needs to be accepted for barrier 8?

_____

What skills could be useful for barrier 8?

_____

Committed action for barrier 8:

_____

Angela's committed action plans for some of her barriers

Barrier 1: You have dropped out of your degree before. What makes you think you will make it now?

Acceptance for barrier 1: *I need to accept the memories and difficult feelings that I experienced previously when I dropped out of my degree.*

Skills for barrier 1: *I can be mindful of these memories and carry them with me while focusing on the present moment.*

Committed action for barrier 1: *I will call the registration office tomorrow morning.*

Barrier 2: You know you will not last for a whole lecture if it's too long. Are you going to embarrass yourself again by leaving in the middle of it?

Acceptance for barrier 2: *I need to accept my bodily sensations while I am in a lecture and also my feelings of embarrassment if I need to go to the loo.*

Skills for barrier 2: *In my mindfulness practice I have faced physical discomfort many times, so I know I can be mindful of what is going on with my belly and still remain in the situation. If I need to get up I can also repeat the word 'embarrassed' 100 times and see it for what it is: a word.*

Committed action for barrier 2: *Get in touch with one of my old lecturers to see if I can sit in on a lecture while I am waiting to restart my studies.*

Barrier 3: How do you expect to get a job if you don't even have your qualifications yet?

Acceptance for barrier 3: *I need to accept that some employers will refuse my applications for lack of experience or qualifications.*

Skills for barrier 3: *I can write my fear on a piece of paper and carry it around with me in my wallet every time I go for an interview.*

Committed action for barrier 3: *I can do some voluntary work to get some more experience while I am trying to get a job. I will continue to apply for the jobs that interest me.*

Barrier 4: Why should you be the one making the effort to call your parents? They never call you!

Acceptance for barrier 4: *I am willing to accept that my parents may not show an interest in me in the way that I would like them to.*

Skills for barrier 4: *From my observer seat I can notice that this 'lack of interest' from my parents is my evaluation of how they act. From my observer seat I can also be open to the feeling of being hurt, knowing it will come and go, and without being overwhelmed by it.*

Committed action for barrier 4: *I will continue to call my parents and I will also ask them if they can show their interest in me in a way that would be more visible to me, like calling me sometimes.*

Barrier 4.1: I will never be able to ask this from my parents. I'm afraid I will feel too embarrassed to do it and that they will think I'm too needy.

Acceptance for barrier 4.1: *I am willing to feel embarrassed and to have the thought that they think I'm needy and still ask them to telephone me at the weekend.*

Skills for barrier 4.1: *I can thank my mind for trying to keep me from having these unpleasant thoughts and feelings. I can put them on the side of one of the buses while using my buses-on-the-street exercise.*

Committed action for barrier 4.1: *When I call my parents next Wednesday I will tell them about how important it is to me that they call me sometimes.*

Barrier 5: You have tried eating your five serves of fruit and vegetables a day before and you didn't last more than a week. It's not going to be different this time.

Acceptance for barrier 5: *I need to accept my difficulties in making the choice of eating healthily.*

Skills for barrier 5: *I can make a committed action plan for my meals. I can embrace my own disappointment if I fail and continue to commit to my plan every day.*

Committed action for barrier 5: *I will build my meal commitment plan right now.*

We hope these exercises and Angela's examples help you deal with the barriers that will come your way on your path towards a valued life. As you can see, the techniques you have learned in this book for accepting your IBS can also be used to deal with all sorts of life barriers. You can also see that sometimes dealing with one barrier brings another one up (like Angela's fourth barrier), and that this one too can be dealt with using your new skills.

Before we conclude this book it is important to address one last thing: the role of other people in this process of change you are going through.

My support team

Getting help from the people who surround you is one of the most rewarding *and* difficult tasks that you could benefit from engaging in.

As you make your choices and start moving in a direction that is consistent with your values, this will be picked up by the people around you. Being able to tell them what is going on for you and having them support you in your actions can help strengthen your choices. Most of the time these people will sense the changes within you and will be able to experience a more vital and complete version of you, and this will naturally draw them closer to support you.

But in other cases, the changes you are bringing about for yourself can be hard on other people, especially if your old actions are ingrained in the relationships you have with these people. For example, suppose that due to your IBS you were staying home most of the time and that by doing so you were also keeping a bedridden relative company. Although being able to go out and live the life you want to live would be a great change for you, it might not be for the person who is left at home. In the long run this person would probably see that this change is for the best, but in the short run it may be very difficult.

The next exercise will help you deal with these situations.

Exercise: Building a support team

Try to see how the changes you are introducing in your life will affect the people who matter to you. It could be your partner, family, friends or co-workers. Jot down the ways you think living according to your values might impact their lives. (Feel free to make a copy of this page if you need more space.)

Who will be affected by my changes and how?

1. _____

_____

_____

2. _____

_____

_____

3. _____

_____

_____

4. _____

_____

_____

5. _____

_____

_____

Now think of the ways these people might react to the changes in your life, and jot them down.

How will they react?

1. _____

_____

2. _____

_____

3. _____

_____

4. _____

_____

5. _____

_____

Finally, think about the ways you could commit to helping those around you understand what these changes are all about, and jot them down.

_____

_____

_____

_____

_____

_____

This exercise will help you foresee difficult reactions from people around you when you move in your valued direction. Recognising the discomfort your changes might bring to others is preferable to leaving them to try to figure out what is going on with you. Communicating your changes can be a delicate art, and being mindful of some aspects while you do it can help you and those closest to you. Consider the following tips:

1. Be clear about the values behind your changes. Let the other person know what it is that is motivating you.

2. Be clear about how the changes you are making link with your values. For example, you might say to a friend you haven't seen in a while: 'I'm going to start calling you to go out more often because I value your company, and I value being able to be there for you.'

3. Once you make a commitment to an action, invite others to share your path so they can experience your increased vitality. For example, if you commit to going to the gym to exercise, invite someone who is important to you to come along.

4. Make room for people's reactions, whether they are positive or negative — especially the latter. Use defusion, mindfulness and acceptance to carry others' reactions while still moving in your valued direction.

Staying committed!

We have been on a long journey in these nine chapters. Through this journey you have learned many skills that can help you live with IBS instead of living a life dictated by IBS. The concepts we visited all come down to the two actions that constitute the core of the approach: acceptance and committed action. By now you probably have a good understanding of the power that these actions can give you: the power to live.

Endnotes

Chapter 1

1 Longstreth, G.F. et al., 2006, 'Functional bowel disorders', *Gastroenterology*, 130(5), pp. 1480–91.
2 Spiller, R. et al., 2007, 'Guidelines on the irritable bowel syndrome: mechanisms and practical management', *Gut*, 56(12), pp. 1770–98.
3 Spiller, R. et al., 2007, 'Guidelines on the irritable bowel syndrome: mechanisms and practical management', *Gut*, 56(12), pp. 1770–98.

Chapter 3

1 See for example: Ruiz, F.J., 2010, 'A Review of Acceptance and Commitment Therapy (ACT) Empirical Evidence: Correlational, Experimental Psychopathology, Component and Outcome Studies', *International Journal of Psychology and Psychological Therapy*, 10(1), pp. 125–162.
2 Corney, R. H., & Stanton, R.,1990, 'Physical symptoms severity, psychological social dysfunction in a series of outpatients with irritable bowel syndrome', *Journal of Psychosomatic Research*, 34(5), pp. 483–491.

Chapter 5

1 See also: Chapter 7 (p. 87) of Hayes, S.C. & Smith, S., 2005, *Get out of your mind and into your life*, New Harbinger, Oakland.

Chapter 9

1 These dartboards are adapted from p. 139 of Dahl, J. & Lundgren, T., 2006, *Living Beyond Your Pain — Using Acceptance and Commitment Therapy to Ease Chronic Pain*, New Harbinger, Oakland.

Appendix

On the following pages are several blank examples of the forms included in this book, for you to photocopy and complete as required. These forms can also be downloaded in PDF form from the websites listed below.

In addition, an audio track for the exercises in this book is available as both a CD and for download.

For further information and links, please visit:

www.betterlivingwithibs.com
or
www.exislepublishing.com

WHAT DID I FEEL?

Examples of emotions: *I felt ... angry, despaired, ashamed, anxious, frustrated, miserable, guilty, nervous, irritated, gloomy, humiliated, tense, aggressive, mournful, blameworthy, worried, disgusted.*

I felt _____ when _____

_____

I felt _____ when _____

_____

I felt _____ when _____

_____

I felt _____ when _____

_____

I felt _____ when _____

_____

I felt _____ when _____

_____

I felt _____ when _____

_____

I felt _____ when _____

_____

I felt _____ when _____

_____

I felt _____ when _____

WHAT DID I EXPERIENCE? WHAT DID I DO?				
Situation	Symptoms	Feelings/ emotions	Thoughts	What did I do?

Exercise: What is avoidance costing you?

Situation	Experience avoided (symptom, thought, feeling)	Short-term effect	Long-term effect	Long-term effect on quality of life

Exercise: What is avoidance costing you?

Situation	Experience avoided (symptom, thought, feeling)	Short-term effect	Long-term effect	Long-term effect on quality of life

FUSION DIARY			
Time	Situation	Thoughts (memory, prediction, evaluation, self-definition or rule)	Actions the thoughts lead to
1 am			
2 am			
3 am			
4 am			
5 am			
6 am			
7 am			
8 am			
9 am			
10 am			
11 am			
12 am			

Time	Situation	Thoughts (memory, prediction, evaluation, self-definition or rule)	Actions the thoughts lead to
1 pm			
2 pm			
3 pm			
4 pm			
5 pm			
6 pm			
7 pm			
8 pm			
9 pm			
10 pm			
11 pm			
12 pm			

FUSION DIARY			
Time	Situation	Thoughts (memory, prediction, evaluation, self-definition or rule)	Actions the thoughts lead to
1 am			
2 am			
3 am			
4 am			
5 am			
6 am			
7 am			
8 am			
9 am			
10 am			
11 am			
12 am			

Time	Situation	Thoughts (memory, prediction, evaluation, self-definition or rule)	Actions the thoughts lead to
1 pm			
2 pm			
3 pm			
4 pm			
5 pm			
6 pm			
7 pm			
8 pm			
9 pm			
10 pm			
11 pm			
12 pm			

FUSION DIARY			
Time	Situation	Thoughts (memory, prediction, evaluation, self-definition or rule)	Actions the thoughts lead to
1 am			
2 am			
3 am			
4 am			
5 am			
6 am			
7 am			
8 am			
9 am			
10 am			
11 am			
12 am			

Time	Situation	Thoughts (memory, prediction, evaluation, self-definition or rule)	Actions the thoughts lead to
1 pm			
2 pm			
3 pm			
4 pm			
5 pm			
6 pm			
7 pm			
8 pm			
9 pm			
10 pm			
11 pm			
12 pm			

Difficult situations diary

What was the situation?

_____
_____
_____

What difficult experiences came up before and during your engagement with this situation (such as bodily sensations, feelings, thoughts)?

_____
_____
_____

What was your mind telling you about all this?

_____
_____
_____
_____

What skills (defusion, mindfulness or others) did you use to accept the situation? How did they work?

_____
_____
_____
_____

Could you improve the use of these skills in the future to be more successful in your acceptance? If yes, how?

_____
_____
_____
_____

Difficult situations diary

What was the situation?

_____

_____

_____

What difficult experiences came up before and during your engagement with this situation (such as bodily sensations, feelings, thoughts)?

_____

_____

_____

What was your mind telling you about all this?

_____

_____

_____

_____

What skills (defusion, mindfulness or others) did you use to accept the situation? How did they work?

_____

_____

_____

_____

Could you improve the use of these skills in the future to be more successful in your acceptance? If yes, how?

_____

_____

_____

_____

Difficult situations diary

What was the situation?

_____

_____

_____

What difficult experiences came up before and during your engagement with this situation (such as bodily sensations, feelings, thoughts)?

_____

_____

_____

What was your mind telling you about all this?

_____

_____

_____

_____

What skills (defusion, mindfulness or others) did you use to accept the situation? How did they work?

_____

_____

_____

_____

Could you improve the use of these skills in the future to be more successful in your acceptance? If yes, how?

_____

_____

_____

_____

Difficult situations diary

What was the situation?

_____

_____

_____

What difficult experiences came up before and during your engagement with this situation (such as bodily sensations, feelings, thoughts)?

_____

_____

_____

What was your mind telling you about all this?

_____

_____

_____

_____

What skills (defusion, mindfulness or others) did you use to accept the situation? How did they work?

_____

_____

_____

_____

Could you improve the use of these skills in the future to be more successful in your acceptance? If yes, how?

_____

_____

_____

_____

Commitment diary

Day: __/__/__

The value I want to pursue is:

_____

_____

_____

What I have been doing that is inconsistent with my value is:

_____

_____

_____

_____

This has cost me (for example, relationships, health, time, money, distress):

_____

_____

_____

_____

The goal I want to achieve is:

_____

_____

_____

_____

I commit to take the following actions in the following circumstances:

_____

_____

_____

_____

In order to perform my valued action I am willing to make room for the following *sensations in my body*:

_____

_____

_____

_____

In order to perform my valued action I am willing to make room for the following *thoughts or images*:

_____

_____

_____

_____

In order to perform my valued action I am willing to make room for the following *feelings or emotions*:

_____

_____

_____

_____

In order to perform my valued action I am willing to make room for the following *urges to avoid* :

_____

_____

_____

_____

Commitment diary

Day: __/__/__

The value I want to pursue is:

_____

_____

_____

What I have been doing that is inconsistent with my value is:

_____

_____

_____

_____

This has cost me (for example, relationships, health, time, money, distress):

_____

_____

_____

_____

The goal I want to achieve is:

_____

_____

_____

_____

I commit to take the following actions in the following circumstances:

_____

_____

_____

_____

In order to perform my valued action I am willing to make room for the following *sensations in my body*:

_____

_____

_____

_____

In order to perform my valued action I am willing to make room for the following *thoughts or images*:

_____

_____

_____

_____

In order to perform my valued action I am willing to make room for the following *feelings or emotions*:

_____

_____

_____

_____

In order to perform my valued action I am willing to make room for the following *urges to avoid* :

_____

_____

_____

_____

Commitment diary

Day: __/__/__

The value I want to pursue is:

_____

_____

_____

What I have been doing that is inconsistent with my value is:

_____

_____

_____

_____

This has cost me (for example, relationships, health, time, money, distress):

_____

_____

_____

_____

The goal I want to achieve is:

_____

_____

_____

_____

I commit to take the following actions in the following circumstances:

_____

_____

_____

_____

Appendix

In order to perform my valued action I am willing to make room for the following *sensations in my body*:

_____

_____

_____

_____

In order to perform my valued action I am willing to make room for the following *thoughts or images*:

_____

_____

_____

_____

In order to perform my valued action I am willing to make room for the following *feelings or emotions*:

_____

_____

_____

_____

In order to perform my valued action I am willing to make room for the following *urges to avoid* :

_____

_____

_____

_____

Commitment diary

Day: __/__/__

The value I want to pursue is:

_____

_____

_____

What I have been doing that is inconsistent with my value is:

_____

_____

_____

_____

This has cost me (for example, relationships, health, time, money, distress):

_____

_____

_____

_____

The goal I want to achieve is:

_____

_____

_____

_____

I commit to take the following actions in the following circumstances:

_____

_____

_____

_____

In order to perform my valued action I am willing to make room for the following *sensations in my body*:

_____

_____

_____

_____

In order to perform my valued action I am willing to make room for the following *thoughts or images*:

_____

_____

_____

_____

In order to perform my valued action I am willing to make room for the following *feelings or emotions*:

_____

_____

_____

_____

In order to perform my valued action I am willing to make room for the following *urges to avoid* :

_____

_____

_____

_____

Index

Index

Printed in Great Britain
by Amazon